TEXTBOOK OF
# NEONATAL
# ULTRASOUND

# TEXTBOOK OF
# NEONATAL
# ULTRASOUND

EDITED BY

## Jack O. Haller MD

State University of New York
Health Science Center at Brooklyn

## The Parthenon Publishing Group
International Publishers in Medicine, Science & Technology

NEW YORK                                      LONDON

**Library of Congress Cataloging-in-Publication Data**
Textbook of Neonatal Ultrasound / edited by Jack O.
  Haller.
        p.   cm
        Includes bibliographical references and index.
        ISBN 1-85070-902-5
        1. Infants — Diseases — Diagnosis.   2. Diagnosis,
Ultrasonic. I. Haller, Jack O. (Jack Oliver), 1944–
        [DNLM: 1. Infant, Newborn, Diseases —
Diagnosis.   2. Infant, Newborn, Diseases —
Ultrasonography.  WS 421 T355 1998]
RJ51.D5T49   1998
618.92'007543—dc21
DNLM/DLC
for Library of Congress                    97-47603
                                                CIP


**British Library Cataloguing in Publication Data**
Textbook of neonatal ultrasound
    1. Infants (Newborn) — Diseases — Diagnosis,
    2. Diagnosis, Ultrasonic
    I. Haller, Jack O.
    618.9'2'007543

ISBN 1-85070-902-5

Published in the USA by
The Parthenon Publishing Group Inc.
One Blue Hill Plaza
Pearl River
New York 10965, USA


Published in the UK and Europe by
The Parthenon Publishing Group Ltd.
Casterton Hall, Carnforth
Lancs. LA6 2LA, UK


Copyright © 1998 Parthenon Publishing Group

First published 1998

Typeset by Speedlith, Manchester, UK
Printed and bound by The Bath Press, Bath, UK

# Contents

# List of contributors

**Sam T. Auringer**
Department of Radiology
Wake Forest University
Bowman Gray School of Medicine
Medical Center Boulevard
Winston-Salem, NC 27157-1088
USA

**Kathleen A. Barry**
Department of Diagnostic Radiology
William Beaumont Hospital
Royal Oak, MI 48073-6769
USA

**Alexander A. Cacciarelli**
Department of Diagnostic Radiology
William Beaumont Hospital
Royal Oak, MI 48073-6769
USA

**Harris L. Cohen**
Department of Radiology
State University of New York
Health Science Center at Brooklyn
450 Clarkson Avenue, Box 1208
Brooklyn, NY 11203
USA

**Susan C.D. Comerci**
Department of Radiology
University of Rochester Medical Center
601 Elmwood Avenue
Rochester, NY 14642-8648
USA

**Michael A. Cook**
Department of Radiology
St. Luke's Roosevelt Hospital Center
Columbia University College of Physicians & Surgeons
New York, NY 10025
USA

**Michael A. DiPietro**
Department of Radiology
1500 East Medical Center Drive
University of Michigan Medical Center
Ann Arbor, MI 48109-0252
USA

**Megan K. Dishop**
Department of Pathology
University of Kentucky Medical Center
Lexington, KY 40502
USA

**Kimberly A. Garver**
Department of Radiology
University of Michigan Medical Center
Ann Arbor, MI 48109-0252
USA

**Jack O. Haller**
Department of Radiology
State University of New York
Health Science Center at Brooklyn
450 Clarkson Avenue, Box 1208
Brooklyn, NY 11203
USA

**S. Zafar H. Jafri**
Department of Diagnostic Radiology
William Beaumont Hospital
Royal Oak, MI 48073-6769
USA

**John C. Leonidas**
Department of Radiology
Schneider Children's Hospital
170-05 76th Avenue
New Hyde Park, NY 11042
USA

**Terry L. Levin**
Department of Radiology
St. Agnes Hospital
305 North Street
White Plains, NY 10605
USA

**Rona J. Orentlicher**
Department of Radiology
State University of New York
Health Science Center at Brooklyn
450 Clarkson Avenue, Box 1208
Brooklyn, NY 11203
USA

**Faridali G. Ramji**
Department of Radiology
Scottish Rite Children's Medical Center
1001 Johnson Ferry Road, NE
Altlanta, GA 30342
USA

**Carrie Ruzal-Shapiro**
Department of Radiology
Babies Hospital
3975 Broadway
New York, NY 10032
USA

**Sandra Schmahmann**
Department of Radiology
Long Island College Hospital
320 Henry Street
Brooklyn, NY
USA

**Joseph M. Silva**
Department of Diagnostic Radiology
Wayne State University
Detroit, MI 48201
USA

**Sudha P. Singh**
Department of Radiology
Schneider Children's Hospital
170-05 76th Avenue
New Hyde Park, NY 11042
USA

**Thomas L. Slovis**
Department of Pediatric Imaging
Children's Hospital of Michigan
3901 Beaubien Boulevard
Detroit, MI 48201
USA

**Thomas E. Sumner**
Department of Radiology
Wake Forest University
Bowman Gray School of Medicine
Medical Center Boulevard
Winston-Salem, NC 27157-1088
USA

**Roger S. Yang**
Department of Radiology
State University of New York
Health Science Center at Brooklyn
450 Clarkson Avenue, Box 1208
Brooklyn, NY 11203
USA

# Foreword

As Editor of this text I have asked my friends, who are all superb pediatric radiologists in major medical centers, to contribute in areas of their expertise. These individuals have had many years of dedicated service to the care and diagnosis of neonatal conditions and many have developed an expertise in that area of speciality. It is to their expertise that I have sought their authorship.

This is a book for two particular audiences. First, it is intended to provide those concerned with the care and treatment of the neonate and young infant with an up-to-date text on the ultrasound manifestations of neonatal disease. Second, it is intended for those concerned with imaging the neonate, i.e. sonographers and radiologists, who rely on ultrasound to diagnose many of the neonatal conditions.

The book does not include echocardiography which really requires a text of its own.

It is my hope that the reader will enjoy this text and that it will prove useful in the day-to-day joy of taking care of the newborn.

Jack O. Haller

# Dedication and acknowledgments

This book is dedicated to my Chairman of 22 years, Joshua A. Becker, M.D., who has supported, encouraged, and provided me with a superb academic environment that allows projects such as this one to be completed. He is the complete scholar, administrator and friend.

I want to thank Gloria Jorge and Barbara Roseman for their contributions to the technical aspects of this manuscript. Also, my colleagues Harris Cohen, M.D. and Rona Orentlicher, M.D. without whom I would not have had the time to complete this work.

# Normal neonatal head ultrasound

1

*Faridali G. Ramji and Thomas L. Slovis*

Major technological advances have occurred since the late 1950s when ultrasound was first utilized by Leksell in the assessment of intracranial contents[1]. The amplitude mode (A-mode) scanning and static gray scale imaging are of only historical interest. The linear array units with large transducers have now been replaced by sector and linear, high frequency, small head transducers that comfortably fit over the fontanelle. The use of water baths and stand-off pads has been replaced by application of standard direct contact coupling gel used for all ultrasound scanning. The patient, who is often premature and in distress, is scanned by portable units brought to the nursery. The examination time has shortened and, in experienced hands, takes 5 to 10 minutes[2]. The resolution of images since Leksell's use of ultrasound in 1956 (A-mode sonography[1]), and the pioneering work of Kossoff and colleagues[3], and Garrett and colleagues[4] on ultrasound of the normal and hydrocephalic neonatal brain have markedly improved with the real-time gray scale imaging[5-43]. The inclusion of color and pulsed wave Doppler has added to the versatility of ultrasound in imaging through the cranium[44-55] and the understanding of vascular anatomy of the brain. Ultrasound has the distinct advantage over computed tomography or magnetic resonance imaging in its portability, being inexpensive, and non-invasive without sedation[10,18,19]. This makes it suitable for imaging neonates in intensive care units (NICU or ICU).

## Embryology relevant to neurosonography

The formation of the central nervous system (CNS) in humans is extremely complex[56-59]. An in-depth discussion of its embryology is beyond the scope of this chapter. However, the key processes that lead to normal development are summarized here. Their inclusion and their understanding aids in the understanding of the normal development of the CNS as well as of congenital and developmental anomalies.

### Neurulation (primary and secondary)

Brain development begins with dorsal induction at approximately day 14 post-fertilization with the formation of the neural plate (primary neurulation) on the dorsal aspect of the embryo[56]. At day 21 post-fertilization, the neural folds begin to fuse at its midpoint converting the neural plate into a neural tube. The fusion and closure proceeds like a zipper with the cranial end of the neural tube or anterior neural pore closing on day 24 and the caudal end or posterior neural pore closing at 26 days post-fertilization[56]. The neural tube will give rise to the brain and spinal cord and the hollow portion of the neural tube will be converted into the ventricular system of the brain and the central canal of the spinal cord. Secondary neurulation results from interactions of notochord and mesoderm in formation of the dura, pia, vertebrae, and skull.

### Ventral induction – formation of brain vesicles

In the beginning of the fourth week post-fertilization, the cranial end of the neural tube undergoes expansion, flexion, and fusion of the neural pores giving rise to three primary brain vesicles: the forebrain or prosencephalon, the midbrain or mesencephalon, and the hindbrain or rhombencephalon[56] (Figure 1). The rapidly growing embryo, especially at the cranial end, undergoes two ventral flexions resulting in a midbrain or mesencephalic flexure at the region of the future midbrain and the cervical flexure at the junction of the hindbrain and the spinal cord (Figure 2). At about the fifth week, the prosencephalon develops into two vesicles, the telencephalon anterior and the diencephalon posterior (Figures 1 and 2).

### Adult derivatives

Neuronal proliferation, differentiation, histogenesis and cellular migration, as well as neuronal

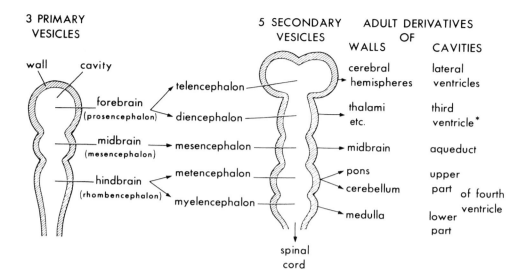

**Figure 1**   Diagrammatic representation of brain vesicles with their wall and cavity and their adult derivatives. *The anterior part of the third ventricle forms from the cavity of the telencephalon but most of the third ventricle is derived from the cavity of the diencephalon.The fourth ventricle results from the cavity of the rhombencephalon and the aqueduct results from the cavity of the mesencephalon. (With permission[56])

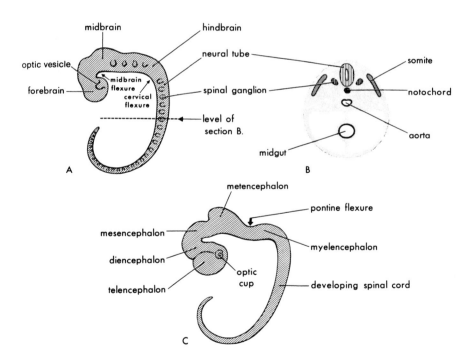

**Figure 2**   Diagrammatic representation of developing brain at the end of the fifth week. A and B depict the rapid growth, expansion, and flexion that occur at the cranial end of the neural tube. The development of the pontine flexure (C) separates the rhombencephalon into its two components, metencephalon superiorly and myelencephalon inferiorly. (With permission[56])

organization, result with subsequent myelination and maturation of the myelin. All are required in formation of the normal CNS. The telencephalon will become the cerebral hemispheres with their lateral ventricles and slit-like third ventricle, and the diencephalon gives rise to the thalamus and hypothalamus and contributes to the formation of neurohypophysis of the pituitary gland[56]. The adenohypophysis or the glandular portion arises from the oral ectoderm or stomoderm. The mesencephalon will give rise to the midbrain. The rhombencephalon gives rise to the myelencephalon and metencephalon. The myelencephalon forms the medulla oblongata, and the metencephalon the pons and the cerebellum.

## Technical considerations, indications and hazards of neurosonography, and anatomy

The sonograms are performed using the highest frequency sector and linear-array transducers (usually 7–10 MHz) which gives optimal resolution of the anatomy. The acoustic windows to intracranial structures are the anterior[24], posterior and posterolateral fontanelles, and the foramen magnum[5] or over other sutures such as the metopic suture[28]. If necessary, scanning through the thin squamosal portion of the temporal bone could be utilized when fontanelles are closed[5,18,24]. Placing the transducer just medial and caudal to the mastoid process allows improved visibility of structures in the posterior fossa[60]. Standard acoustic coupling gel is placed over the surface of the head. The commonly used acoustic window is the anterior fontanelle with images carried out in coronal, modified coronal, sagittal and modified sagittal planes. Imaging is modified because we must scan through a fixed point, such as the anterior fontanelle[6].

Image quality should be maximized and may require the adjusting of many technical parameters. This includes the transmit zone enhancement, depth compensation, persistence, pre- and post-processing adjustments, and the number of focal zones[5]. We obtain both video tape and gray scale hard copy for documentation, but the most recent innovation is the filmless department with all reading from the monitor and storage via optical disk (or tape).

The clinical indications of head ultrasound in the neonate, premature or term, have been summarized in Table 1[2,61]. Although no known deleterious effects have resulted or have been reported from diagnostic ultrasound, nevertheless,

**Table 1** Clinical indications for ultrasonic intracranial evaluation[2,61]

*Premature infants*
In all less than 1500 g or < 32 weeks gestation
Suspected intracranial bleeding
As follow-up to any detected abnormality, i.e. enlarged ventricles, parenchymal injury
Secondary to bleeding
Secondary to hypoxia/apnea

*Premature or full-term infants*
Large or rapidly enlarging head size, or increased intracranial pressure
Seizures
Cranial bruits
Meningomyelocele patient/CNS anomaly
Following central nervous system infection
    subdural collection
    ventriculitis
    parenchymal changes (abscess, other)
Traumatized or asphyxiated infant
Follow-up on surgical procedures or shunt placement (ECMO)
Low Apgar

*Older child*
Through craniotomy site for evaluation of ventricular size

there may be hazards from the procedure of performing the neurosonogram on the premature neonate, and this requires mention[62]. The hazards include inadvertently moving the endotracheal tube, spread of infection due to inadequate cleaning of the transducers and/or the operator's hands, hypothermia may result during the procedure, and bradycardia from application of too much pressure on the fontanelle with the transducer. Precautions suggested include: (1) minimizing head and neck movement, (2) minimizing pressure applied on the fontanelle, (3) using prewarmed coupling gel which is removed after scanning to minimize heat loss due to evaporation, (4) careful handwashing, and (5) wiping the transducer with 70% isopropyl alcohol or 2% alkalinized glutaraldehyde between studies[62].

It is important that every patient's head ultrasound is carried out in a standard manner and the same anatomical landmarks[13] are imaged such that normal and abnormal anatomy can be correlated from one patient to another. This also allows all technologists performing neonatal head ultrasound to be consistent even when one patient is scanned by several technologists during the course of a hospital stay. In the coronal plane we obtain eight ultrasound images, all acquired by radially sweeping the transducer from anterior to posterior cranium (Figure 3). In the sagittal plane there are five images obtained, one in the midline and two in the parasagittal region on each side of the midline (Figure 3). Four additional images are obtained with the linear array transducer, one coronal and three sagittal for improved resolution and detection of small subependymal hemorrhage.

### Scanning in the coronal plane

In the coronal plane, the following images are obtained (Figures 4 and 5).

(1) The transducer is angled forward, anterior to the frontal horn, such that bright echoes result from the orbital roof and ethmoid complex (Figures 4 and 5). The anterior part of the cerebral hemispheres gives fine but low level echoes and the echogenic midline falx oriented vertically in the interhemispheric fissure is demonstrated (Figures 4a and 5). The bony reflective echoes give a 'steer's head' appearance[13] (Figure 4a).

(2) The second coronal plane is slightly posterior to the first plane such that the 'steer's head' changes to a 'mask' appearance[13] (Figure 4b). This results from the lesser wing of the sphenoid giving rise to the echogenic upper portion of the mask; the lower portions of the mask are reflections resulting from the greater wings of the sphenoid forming the anterior floor of the temporal fossa (Figure 4b). The central portions of the mask are formed by dense echoes resulting from the planum sphenoidale. The echogenic falx in the interhemispheric fissure forms a prominent vertical landmark where the anterior cerebral artery pulsations are noted. Short horizontal echoes arising from the brain surface are visible just off the midline and, of these, the most prominent is that resulting from the cingulate sulcus with the cingulate gyrus just below it. The slit-like semi-lunar shaped hypoechoic regions on either side of midline are the frontal horn of the lateral ventricles with the caudate nucleus abutting and indenting each lateral wall (Figure 5).

(3) The third coronal landmark is the sylvian fissure between the frontal lobe and the temporal lobe which appear as 'Y' shaped[13] (Figures 4 and 5). The echogenicity is not as pronounced as bone and results from the combination of pulsating branches of the middle cerebral artery and the

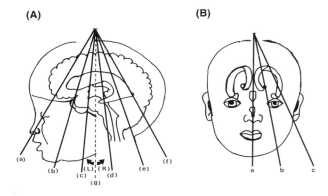

**Figure 3** Planes of transfontanelle cranial ultrasound. (A) coronal sections: plane (a) anteriorly to the frontal horn of the lateral ventricles. Plane (b) through the frontal horn of the lateral ventricles. Plane (c) at or just anterior to the foramen of Monro. Plane (d) section just posterior to the foramen of Monro. Plane (e) through the body of the lateral ventricles and plane (f) through the atria or trigone of the lateral ventricles. Plane (g) are angled coronal scans on each side at the level of the foramen of Monro and arrows indicate angulation left (L) or right (R). (B) sagittal sections: plane (a) sagittal plane in the midline. Plane (b) and (c) are 15° and 30° parasagittal angulation, respectively. (Reprinted with permission[2,13])

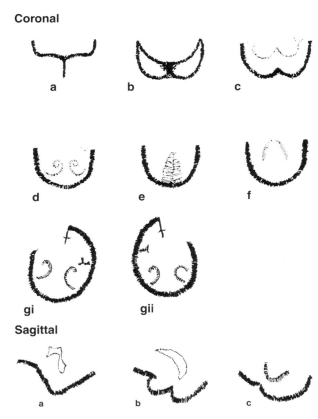

**Figure 4** Diagrammatic representation of bony landmarks seen during the performance of a transcranial ultrasound in the coronal and sagittal planes. The bony and parenchymal features represented are referred to in the relevant text and sonographic planes are depicted in Figure 3. gi, angulation to left; gii, angulation to right. (Modified with permission[13])

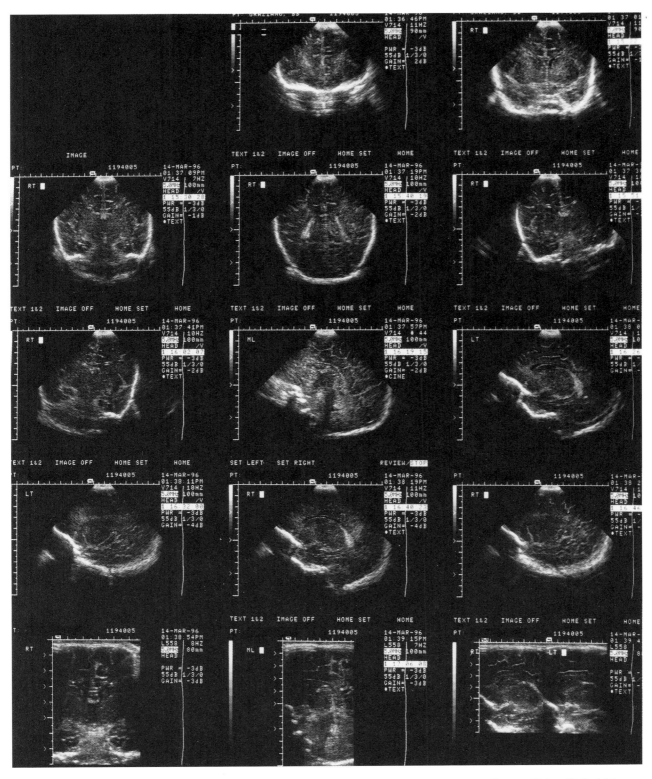

**Figure 5**   A standard head ultrasound. The first blank square is the patient's relevant data and the clinical history. This is followed by six coronal images using a sector transducer, two of which are in the angled coronal planes. The five sagittal images using sector transducer are then acquired. This is followed by obtaining one in the coronal and three in the sagittal planes using a high resolution linear transducer specifically in the midline and at the level of the caudothalamic grooves (the last picture is a composite dual image at each caudothalamic groove). Performing the sonogram in this manner allows for one film consisting of all the patient data plus 14 images. (See Figure 19 for details of individual images)

collagen of the leptomeninges. The appearance of the sylvian fissure may serve as a clue to gestational age and will be discussed later. This ultrasound image is at or just anterior to the foramen of Monro. The slit-like anechoic frontal horns of the lateral ventricles are again visualized but situated slightly more posterior than on the previous image and have more of a 'boomerang' shape than the semi-lunar shape[13] (Figure 5). In the midline between the ventricles lies the echogenic septum pellucidum and, often in the premie with fluid between the two walls, the anechoic cavum septum pellucidum. Inferolateral to the frontal horn lies the head of the caudate nucleus which is of medium echogenicity. Lateral to the caudate are the anterior limb of the internal capsule and the lentiform nucleus (comprised of globus pallidus medially and putamen laterally). In the near field above the roof of the frontal horns is the genu of the corpus callosum, which is composed of homogeneously packed axons and appears hypoechoic except at its surface which is echogenic due to pial tissue. In the midfield below the septum pellucidum is the slit-like foramen of Monro.

(4) This section is just posterior to the foramen of Monro and, when there are no abnormalities identified, could be combined with the image prior to it. However, the image behind the foramen of Monro shows the anechoic bodies of the lateral ventricle and the echogenic choroid plexus lie on the floor of the ventricle. The third ventricle may not be visible in the coronal plane or it may appear as a slit-like structure in the midline below the lateral ventricle. On either side of the third ventricle is the thalamus, which is of medium echogenicity. Further lateral are the medial extensions of the sylvian fissure. Prominent landmarks on this image in the far field are the C-shaped structures composed of parahippocampal gyrus and the medial gyrus of the temporal lobe (Figure 4d). In the midline between the temporal lobes are the cerebral peduncles. A normal temporal horn of the lateral ventricle is rarely seen on this plane[19].

(5) Further posterior angulation results in a landmark composed of an echogenic inverted 'V' formed by the cerebellum medially and the tentorium laterally[13] (Figure 4e). The sonolucent normal lateral ventricle is not prominent but outlines the echogenic choroid plexus. In the midline the quadrigeminal plate cistern may be visible as a small echogenic area, containing vessels and leptomeninges.

(6) The sixth image is posterior to the previous image. The very bright echoes in the far field are

from the calvarium. In the midfield, the glomus of choroid plexus appear as divergent echogenic bands located in the trigone of the lateral ventricle (Figures 4 and 5). Around the choroid may be the anechoic cerebrospinal fluid (CSF) of the lateral ventricle but generally the choroid plexus on this image fills the lateral ventricle.

(7) Coronal angled images are routinely obtained and are quite helpful in detecting extra-axial fluid over convexities of the brain. This view is performed by obtaining an image on each side with the transducer in the coronal plane but angled to the left or right at the level of the foramen of Monro (Figures 3, 4 and 5). These images can be acquired at any time in the study. One additional image is obtained in the coronal plane through the foramen of Monro with a linear array transducer. The linear transducer provides better resolution (see Figures 4 and 5), especially for detecting subtle bleeds.

## Scanning in the sagittal plane

In the sagittal plane, the following images are routinely obtained (Figures 4 and 5).

(1) The midline sagittal image is one of the most important, especially in ruling out any congenital anatomical abnormalities and in defining the posterior fossa. The superior sagittal sinus, which is the most superior portion of the falx cerebri, can be assessed as it lies under the anterior fontanelle. Visualization requires color Doppler and this will be addressed later with vascular anatomy. The cingulate gyrus is identified and is limited superiorly by the cingulate sulcus and inferiorly by the callosal sulcus (Figure 5). The gyrus consists of hypoechoic gray matter and slightly echogenic white matter centrally. The corpus callosum is a hypoechoic structure, the thickness of which may vary with age. The cavum septum pellucidum is seen below the corpus callosum in most premature infants. The massa intermedia or the thalamic adhesion (intrathalamic connection) and the foramen of Monro are seen easily. The third ventricle is best seen on this image with its chiasmatic and infundibular recesses anteriorly and pineal and habenular recesses posteriorly. Further inferior and posterior are the aqueduct of Sylvius and posterior fossa with the fourth ventricle. Posterior to the fourth ventricle is the midline cerebellum – the echogenic vermis. The triangular tip of the roof of the fourth ventricle is called the fastigium. The cisterna magna lies posterior and inferior to the cerebellum and should be identified

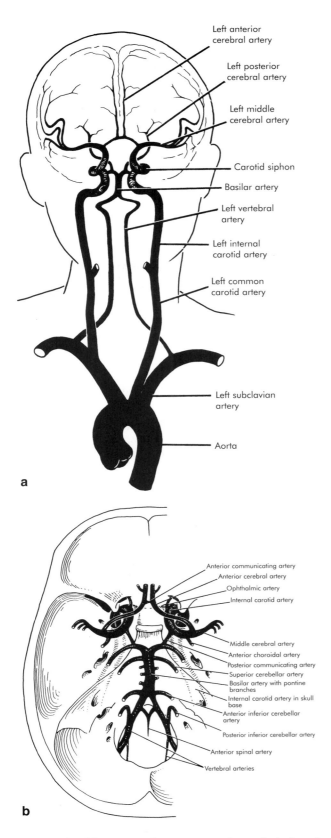

Left anterior
cerebral artery

Left posterior
cerebral artery

Left middle
cerebral artery

Carotid siphon

Basilar artery

Left vertebral
artery

Left internal
carotid artery

Left common
carotid artery

Left subclavian
artery

Aorta

**a**

Anterior communicating artery
Anterior cerebral artery
Ophthalmic artery
Internal carotid artery

Middle cerebral artery
Anterior choroidal artery
Posterior communicating artery
Superior cerebellar artery
Basilar artery with pontine branches
Internal carotid artery in skull base
Anterior inferior cerebellar artery
Posterior inferior cerebellar artery
Anterior spinal artery
Vertebral arteries

**b**

**Figures 6** Diagrammatic representation of circle of Willis[64], (a) and (b)

on all scans. The basilar portion of the brain stem shows increased echoes due to heterogenous texture resulting from multiple long tracks and nuclei seated in the pons and medulla. However, the dorsal portion of the brain stem is relatively hypoechoic due to homogenous longitudinal tracks and diverse nuclei in the midbrain, pons, and the medulla. These three portions of the brainstem are clearly defined posterior to the prepontine cistern. Immediately anterior to the cistern is the basilar artery, and anterior to it the bony clivus is seen as multiple echogenic structures running obliquely from anterior to posterior. The reason for the multiplicity of bony structures apparently relates to the angles the echoes traverse the bone. In the far field posteriorly is the echogenic calvarium (Figures 4 and 5).

(2) The first parasagittal image is angled approximately 15 degrees laterally. The prominent echogenic landmark in the far field is the shape of an omega and corresponds to the floor of the middle cranial fossa where the temporal horn of the lateral ventricle may be seen (Figures 4 and 5). In the midfield are the anechoic lateral ventricles which contain echogenic choroid plexus extending from the floor of the body of the lateral ventricle to its trigone and into the temporal horn. This image is very important in the premature infant as the caudo-thalamic groove, between the head of the caudate and the thalamus, is where hemorrhage may first be visualized[8,26,42].

(3) The second parasagittal image is obtained angling approximately 30 degrees laterally such that it is lateral to the lateral ventricle (Figures 4 and 5). The prominent landmark here is the smooth echogenic curve of the calvarium in the far field. Above this is the echogenic sylvian fissure with pulsating branches of the middle cerebral artery.

Using a linear array transducer, we routinely obtain three additional sagittal images; two of these are through the caudo-thalamic grooves, one image from each side simply to detect subependymal hemorrhage. The third image is through the midline which complements the sector image done earlier. This is for improved resolution and sensitivity, especially for the posterior fossa structures. Altogether, after following this protocol, there will be 15 images. When there are no abnormalities noted, the coronal image (b) and (c) may be combined as a single image through the foramen of Monro thus resulting in one film consisting of 14 images (Figure 5). In the one remaining blank box (first of the 15 boxes on the single sheet of film), the

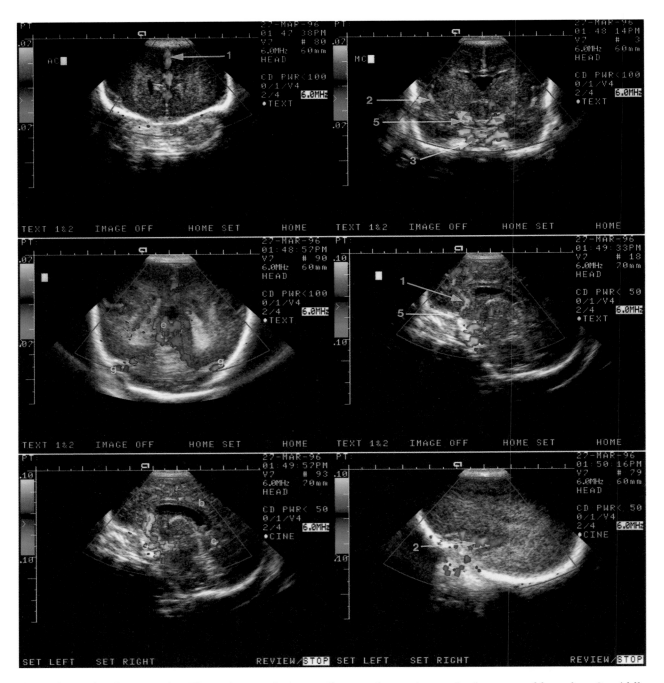

**Figure 7**   Color flow Doppler. The major arteries are easily seen. 1, anterior cerebral artery and branches; 2, middle cerebral artery; 3, posterior cerebral artery; 4, basilar artery; 5, internal carotid artery; 6, pericallosal vessels: a, superior sagittal sinus (SSS); b, inferior sagittal; c, straight sinus; d, vein of Galen; e, internal cerebral vein (paired); f, cortical veins over convexity draining into SSS; g, transverse sinus

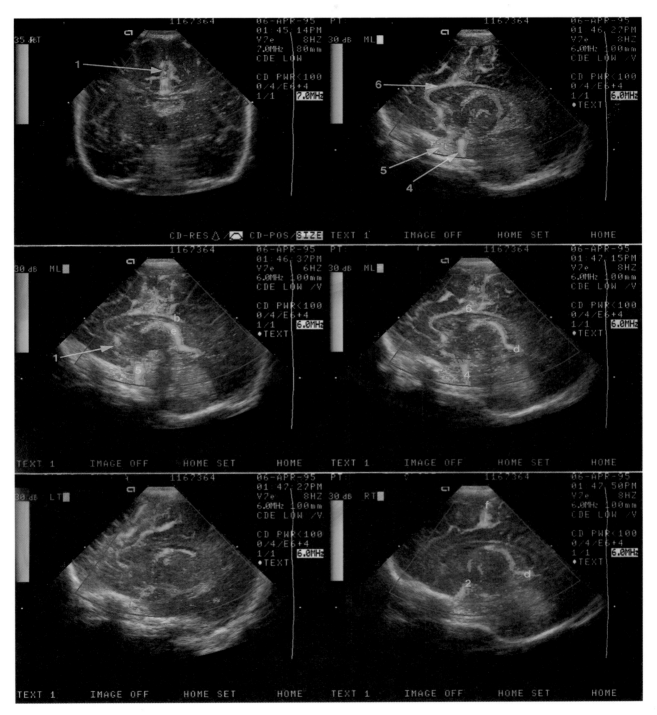

**Figure 8** Power Doppler. Note the greater number of vessels seen. With power Doppler one cannot separate arteries from veins. 1, anterior cerebral artery and branches; 2, middle cerebral artery; 3, posterior cerebral artery; 4, basilar artery; 5, internal carotid artery; 6, pericallosal vessels: a, superior sagittal sinus (SSS); b, inferior sagittal; c, straight sinus; d, vein of Galen; e, internal cerebral vein (paired); f, cortical veins over convexity draining into SSS; g, transverse sinus

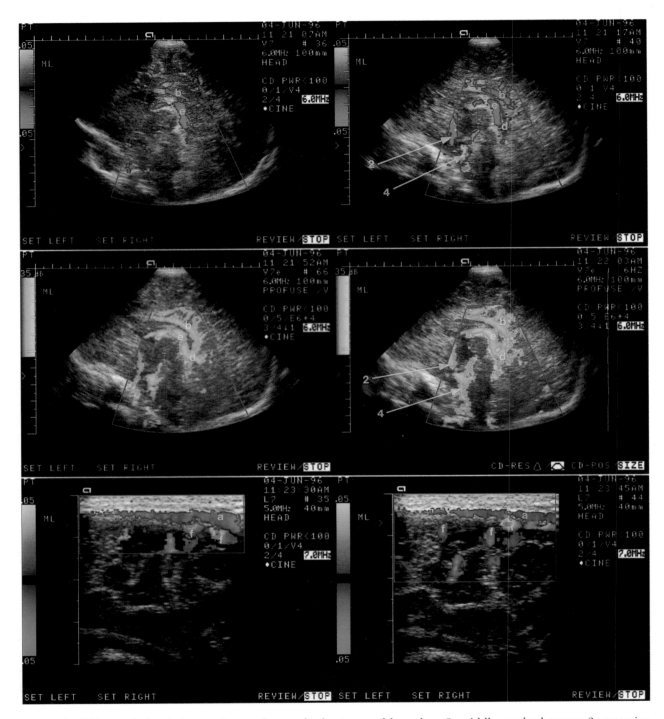

**Figure 9** Veins and dural sinuses. 1, anterior cerebral artery and branches; 2, middle cerebral artery; 3, posterior cerebral artery; 4, basilar artery; 5, internal carotid artery; 6, pericallosal vessels: a, superior sagittal sinus (SSS); b, inferior sagittal; c, straight sinus; d, vein of Galen; e, internal cerebral vein (paired); f, cortical veins over convexity draining into SSS; g, transverse sinus

patient's history is written. As in any other sonographic examination, these standard images are obtained as permanent record, but the entire brain is examined by radially scanning in any plane. However, when an abnormality is seen, more images should be obtained. Note that the individual images in Figure 5 are produced in detail and discussed below (mature brain).

*Vascular anatomy to the brain*

The two pairs of vessels, the internal carotid (ICA) and the vertebral arteries, supply the brain[63,64] (Figure 6 a, b). Each ICA arises from the common carotid artery in the neck approximately at the level of the superior border of the thyroid cartilage. For convenience, the ICA is divided anatomically into four parts: (1) cervical, (2) petrous, (3) cavernous, and (4) cerebral. The cervical portion ascends up in the neck to the base of the skull entering the carotid canal in the petrous part of the temporal bone and thus becoming the petrous portion. The petrous portion passes through the foramen lacerum coursing anteriorly and enters the cavernous sinus, appropriately referred to as the cavernous portion. The cavernous portion of the ICA leaves the cavernous sinus after making a hairpin turn and enters the subarachnoid space.

Each of the vertebral arteries (VA) arises from the first part of the subclavian artery in the root of the neck. It ascends within the transverse foramen of C7–C1 vertebrae and courses posteriorly almost at a right angle, winding around the superior part of the lateral mass of C1. The VA enters the subarachnoid space at the level of the foramen magnum after passing through the atlanto-occipital membrane and the dura. It runs anteriorly along the anterolateral surface of the medulla, uniting with its counterpart from the opposite side to form the basilar artery at the junction of the medulla and pons. The basilar artery courses on the belly of the pons within the prepontine cistern to the superior border of the pons, dividing into the posterior cerebral arteries.

Together the two internal carotid arteries, the horizontal segments of both anterior cerebral arteries, the anterior communicating arteries, the proximal segments of both posterior cerebral arteries, and the two posterior communicating arteries form the cerebral arterial circle, also known as the circle of Willis (Figure 6 a, b). On color Doppler ultrasound using standard technique through the anterior fontanelle, the

major vessels seen are shown in Figures 7–9. These include the cavernous and cerebral portions of the ICA, anterior cerebral artery, posterior cerebral artery, middle cerebral artery and many other branches[44,45] (Figures 7, 8 and 9). Transcranial Doppler through the temporal squamosa allows visualization of the major cerebral vessels[49,50].

The cerebral blood drains through the dural sinuses (Figures 8 and 9) of which the superior sagittal sinus, inferior sagittal sinus, straight sinus, transverse sinus, as well as the cortical veins and vein of Galen could be identified[46] (Figure 9).

Color Doppler energy or amplitude imaging, if available, may be utilized as it has greater sensitivity to detect vessels with less flow. The information depicted comes from the amplitude components of the Doppler echo, not the usual frequency component. The signal is proportional to the number of moving blood cells in each sample volume[48] (Figure 8). The normal pulsation of vessels seen on color Doppler can also be appreciated on standard real-time gray scale and their velocity and quality can be observed on duplex Doppler[55].

## The changing brain with gestation

Characteristic changes occur in brain development and have been recognized on anatomical specimens[65–68]. The development and maturation of various gyri, sulci, and fissures proceed in a recognizable manner. This pattern can also be recognized on the fetal and neonatal head ultrasound and serves as a reliable guide to determination of gestational age[69–73].

The temporal development of cerebral hemispheres are defined by intervals between two and three weeks because this is the minimum duration required for observing any recognizable change on ultrasound[73]. Brain maturation varies slightly from one individual to another as well as from side to side within each individual due to inherent biological variations.

At the end of the first trimester, the brain surface is smooth with no surface sulci[58,73]. This is referred to as the lissencephalic stage[58] (Figure 10). Initial sulcation consists of formation of a shallow groove with widely separated side walls without any branching. This shallow groove deepens into a furrow and the side walls become steeper. The opposing side walls of the gyri facing the sulci progressively lie closer and closer together until they abut and mold each other into a 'parallel' configuration[73] (Figure 10). Individual sulci may join adjacent other developing sulci, or be

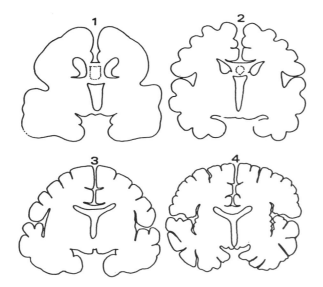

**Figure 10** Diagrammatic representation of four normal stages of gyration: (1) lissencephaly stage, (2) differentiation of primary gyri, (3) deeper infolding brain surface, and (4) the adult pattern. (With permission[58])

displaced by them or simply lie adjacent. The brain between the sulci is called the gyrus and is named accordingly depending on its location and configuration in the lobe of the brain in which it is seated[73].

The sulcal groove initially is a single line with straight ends and these are called primary sulci or sulcus. With time, these deepen to show V-shaped terminations or may show bifid ends[73]. With continual brain maturation and formation of gyri and sulci, there is development of side sulcal branches or secondary sulci which arise from the main sulci. These secondary sulci (initially two) have straight edges and mature to form V-shaped terminations. With further growth, the secondary sulci develop side branches too and these are called tertiary sulci, seen in adults. These very complex changes are clearly visible on the gross specimens of brain from 22–40 weeks gestation[66] (Figure 11).

Early in development the brain is loosely applied against the calvarium; the subarachnoid spaces as well as convexity cisterns surrounding the primary sulci are large. The surface of the gyri is round. The subarachnoid space and convexity cisterns progressively diminish as the gyri grow and the primary sulci form secondary and then tertiary sulci. The gyri get 'squared off'[73].

Sulcal development has been shown to be a reliable index of gestational age of infant and histological maturation[65–73]. Chi and colleagues[67]

sequentially studied the appearance and development of fissures, sulci and gyri on anatomical brain specimens of infants ranging in gestational age from 10 to 44 weeks. The appearance of lateral and medial surfaces of brains from 22 to 40 weeks gestation at intervals of 2 weeks has been provided and reproduced in Figure 11 (courtesy of Professor Katerina Dorovini-Lis, MD).

Murphy and colleagues studied ultrasounds of sulci along the lateral and medial surfaces of the brain, including closure of the opercula to determine brain maturity in terms of gestational age, from 24 weeks to 34 weeks[71] (Table 2). They found that the most reliable sulci noted were: cingulate sulcus, pre- and post-central, superior and inferior temporal sulci, and sequential maturation and infolding of the operculum to form the sylvian fissure (Figure 12). Building on these data, Huang analyzed sonograms of several sulci along the convex and medial surface of the brain and established a criteria for determination of gestational age base on brain maturity[72,73] (Tables 3 and 4). It is important to realize that there may be considerable lag in visualizing certain sulci on ultrasound when compared with anatomical data[72,73] (Table 5).

Twenty-four premature patients were followed sequentially and these data form the illustrations in Figures 13–18. The tables included here are based on ultrasound landmarks and utilize data from references 65–73 (Tables 2–6). The data published have been summarized with details by Naidich and colleagues[73] (Table 5).

*Interhemispheric fissure (longitudinal fissure)*

The interhemispheric fissure is the earliest primary fissure to develop and is present at 8 weeks gestation, beginning anteriorly and proceeding posteriorly. This structure is well defined anatomically and separates the two cerebral hemispheres by 10 weeks gestation. It is important to document the presence of the interhemispheric fissure on neonatal ultrasound to eliminate congenital anomalies, i.e. more severe forms of holoprosencephaly, but this will not give a clue to gestational age as it should be present as a distinct structure on all newborn premies (Figures 13–18).

*Sylvian fissure*

A shallow depression appearing at 14 weeks gestation is seen between the future orbitofrontal

**Table 2** Appearance and increasing complexity of the principal sulci noted in each plane with increasing maturity[71]

| | Midsagittal (midline) | | Tangential (parasagittal) | | Coronal |
|---|---|---|---|---|---|
| 0 | Calcarine and posterior calcarine sulci already present. Absent cingulate sulcus | 0 | Smooth cerebral hemisperes. Lateral sulcus wide open | 0 | Wide open appearance of lateral sulci |
| 1 | Calcarine and posterior calcarine sulci more apparent. First appearance of cingulate sulcus | 1 | Central sulci may appear. Lateral sulcus closing | 1 | Early closure of lateral sulci (apposition of parietal and temporal lobes) |
| 2 | Cingulate sulcus easily visible straight and simple | 2 | Central and postcentral sulci visible. Lateral sulcus closed. First appearance of superior temporal sulcus | 2 | Further closure of lateral sulci |
| 3 | Posterior calcarine and parieto-occipital sulci more compressed. Cingulate sulcus more tortuous, now extending posteriorly | 3 | Lateral sulcus more tortuous with further closure. Superior temporal sulcus more apparent, inferior temporal sulcus now visible | 3 | Lateral sulci now fully closed |
| 4 | Cingulate sulcus more tortuous, now extending posteriorly | 4 | Inferior temporal sulcus more apparent | 4 | Lateral sulci now fully closed and more tortuous, with increase in size of the parietal and temporal lobes |
| 5 | Further posterior extension of cingulate sulcus. Further compression of parieto-occipital and posterior calcarine sulci | 5 | Superior frontal sulcus now visible | | |

Scoring system: 0: 24–25 weeks; 5: 34+ weeks

**Table 3** Ultrasonic landmarks for sulcal maturation[72,73]

| Sulcus/fissure | Early development | Landmark: proportion sulcus is well-defined in |
|---|---|---|
| Parieto-occipital fissure | | All by 24 WG |
| Calcarine sulcus | 75% by 24–25 WG | All by 26–27 WG |
| Cingulate sulcus | | |
|   (A) anterior | 25% by 24–25 WG | |
| | 83% by 26–27 WG | All after 27 WG |
|   (B) entire complete | 10% by 26–27 WG | |
| | 83% by 28–29 WG | All after 29 WG |
|   (C) curvy shape | | After 30 WG |
|   (D) secondary sulci | 27% at 30–31 WG | All after 32–33 WG |
|   (E) tertiary sulci | 50% at 36 WG | |
| Post-central sulcus | 42% by 26–27 WG | All by 28–29 WG |
| Sylvian fissure | | |
|   (covering of insula) | Widely open in all: < 28 WG | Closed in 91% after 29 WG |
| | closed: 25% at 28–29 WG | |
| Inferior temporal sulcus | 17% at 28–29 WG | 91% by 30–31 WG |
| Insular sulci | | |
|   (A) partial | 57% by 32–33 WG | |
|   (B) complete | 67% by 34–35 WG | All at 36 WG |

WG, weeks gestation

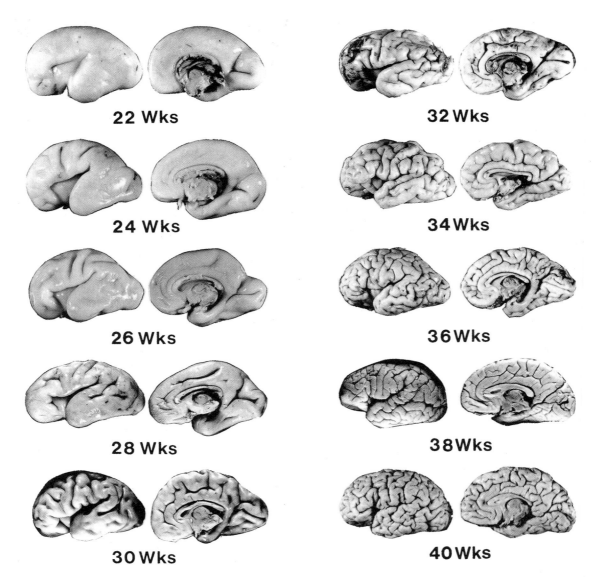

**Figure 11**   Characteristic configuration of fetal brain from 2 to 40 weeks gestation at two week intervals. All brains have been brought to same size. (Reproduced with permission[66])

and the temporal lobe and is the earliest development of the sylvian fissure. The fissure deepens and by 19 weeks gestation the tissue deep to the fissure is defined as the insula. The superior border of the insula is called the circular sulcus and the inferior border is the proper sylvian fissure; these combine to form a single deep fissure (sylvian fissure).

The sonographic appearance of the sylvian fissure on the coronal plane as well as on the angled coronal plane could be a clue as to the gestational age. Before the age of 24 to 26 weeks the insula is exposed and the sylvian fissure is widely open; it begins to close after 28 weeks gestation. It is closed in approximately 91% of

infants after 29 weeks gestation. By 30–31 weeks the insula is completely covered, and by 32–33 weeks partial insular sulci and, beyond 36 weeks, mature insular sulci are visible (Figures 13–18).

*Callosal sulcus*

The callosal sulcus separates the corpus callosum and the overlying cingulate gyrus and appears at 14 weeks gestational age. This is a fairly constant feature on the neurosonogram by 24 weeks gestation. Its presence does not provide a clue to determination of the gestational age.

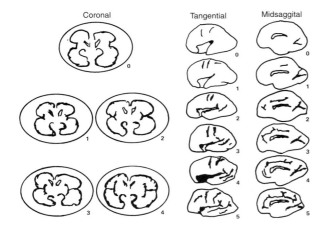

**Figure 12** Anatomical diagrams showing the increasing complexity of the principal sulci noted on each plane with increasing maturity. See Table 2 for explanation of the grading. (With permission[71])

**Table 4** Cortical maturation: ultrasonic landmarks[72,73]

| Weeks of gestation | Ultrasonic landmarks |
|---|---|
| 24–25 | Prominent parieto-occipital sulcus |
| | Early branching calcarine sulcus |
| 26–27 | Matured calcarine sulcus |
| | Anterior cingulate sulcus |
| 28–29 | Whole cingulate sulcus |
| | Post central sulcus |
| | Insula partly covered |
| 30–31 | Insula covered completely |
| | Cingulate sulcus arcs, curves |
| | Inferior temporal sulcus |
| | +/– Secondary cingulate sulci |
| 32–33 | Secondary cingulate sulci |
| | Partial insular sulci |
| 34–35 | Better insular sulci |
| | Maturer secondary sulci |
| | +/– tertiary sulci |
| > 36 | Tertiary sulci |
| | Maturer insular sulci |

### Cingulate sulcus and gyrus

While the cingulate sulcus is present in the anterior frontal lobe by 18 weeks gestation, its visibility on ultrasound may lag behind by 8–9 weeks[72]. Its presence can be documented between 24 and 25 weeks in approximately 25% of infants[72,73] (Tables 5 and 6). The development of the cingulate sulcus proceeds posteriorly and can be seen on ultrasound in the majority of infants by 29 weeks (Figures 13, 14 and 15). After 30 weeks gestation it has a curvy shape, and between 30 and 33 weeks there is development of secondary sulci. After 38 weeks, development of tertiary sulci and multiple sulci could be appreciated (Figure 15). There is no lag in the ultrasound visibility of these secondary and tertiary cingulate sulci[72]. Beyond 38 weeks, the cingulate sulcus has a cobblestone appearance[72,73].

### Olfactory sulcus

The olfactory sulcus appears anatomically at 16 weeks gestation along the inferior aspect of the orbital segment of the frontal lobe and parallels the interhemispheric fissure. Its appearance separates the gyrus rectus located medial to the sulcus from the remainder orbital segment of the frontal lobe. The sulcal groove deepens with progressive gestation and becomes prominent by 25 weeks gestation, and its presence on ultrasound can be

**Table 6** Cingulate sulcus: ultrasound*[70,73]

| Weeks of gestation | Ultrasonic appearance |
|---|---|
| > 24 | Present |
| 28–33 | Continuous |
| 28–34 | First branch |
| 33–38 | Multiple branches |
| 38–40 | Cobblestone |

*Reproduced with permission and modified

**Table 5** Ultrasound display lags behind anatomy[72,73]

| Age of sulcal appearance by ultrasound | Delay from anatomic appearance | Example |
|---|---|---|
| < 28 WG | 8–9 weeks | Calcarine sulcus |
| | | Cingulate sulcus |
| 2 –31 WG | 1–3 weeks | Postcentral sulcus |
| | | Inferior temporal sulcus |
| > 31 WG | None | Secondary and tertiary cingulate sulci |
| | | Insular sulci |

WG, weeks gestation

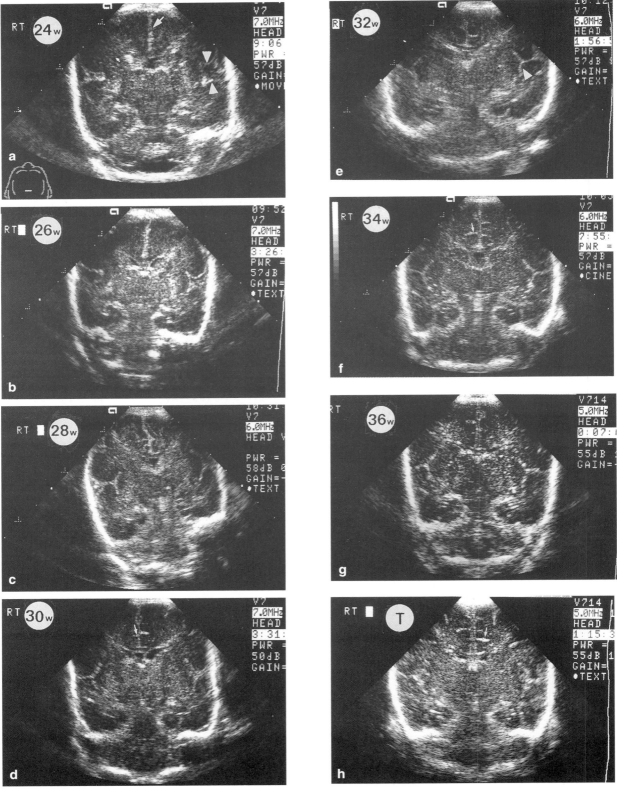

**Figure 13 (a–h)**   Coronal plane through the foramen of Monro at two week intervals. Note that with progressive gestation the sylvian fissure (arrowhead) becomes smaller in size with the opposing walls progressively adhering and the fissures becoming longer and branching. Also note the surface of the brain is smooth at 24 weeks and, with development of gyri and sulci, the brain becomes progressively complex. On either side of the falx cerebri (arrow) the cingulate sulci (small arrow) and the gyrus develop and its sulci deepen with gestation. Gestation time as indicated on each image (T, term)

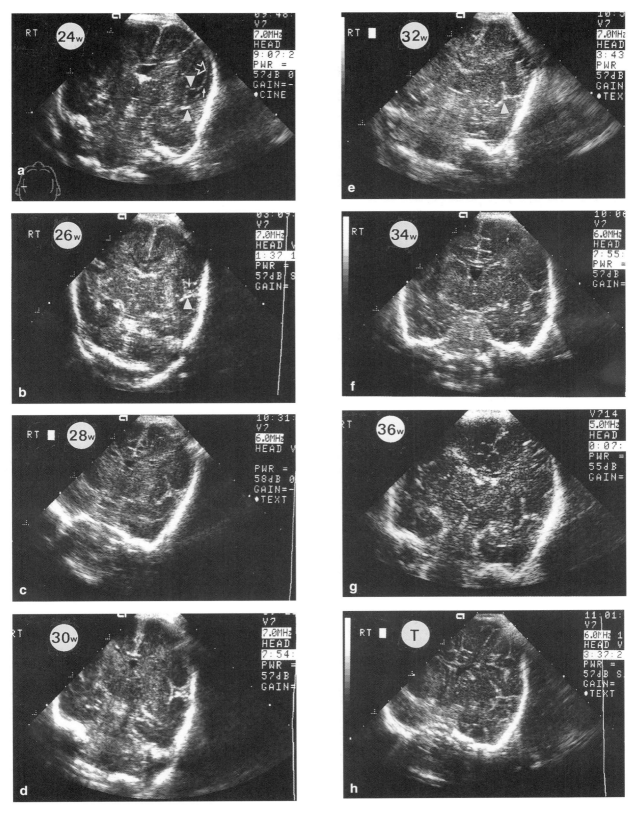

**Figure 14 (a–h)**    Angled coronal ultrasound at two week intervals. Note with progressive gestation the change in appearance of the surface of the brain (open arrow) as well as the sylvian fissure (arrowhead). The subarachnoid space disappears with maturity (small arrow). Gestation time as indicated on each image (T, term)

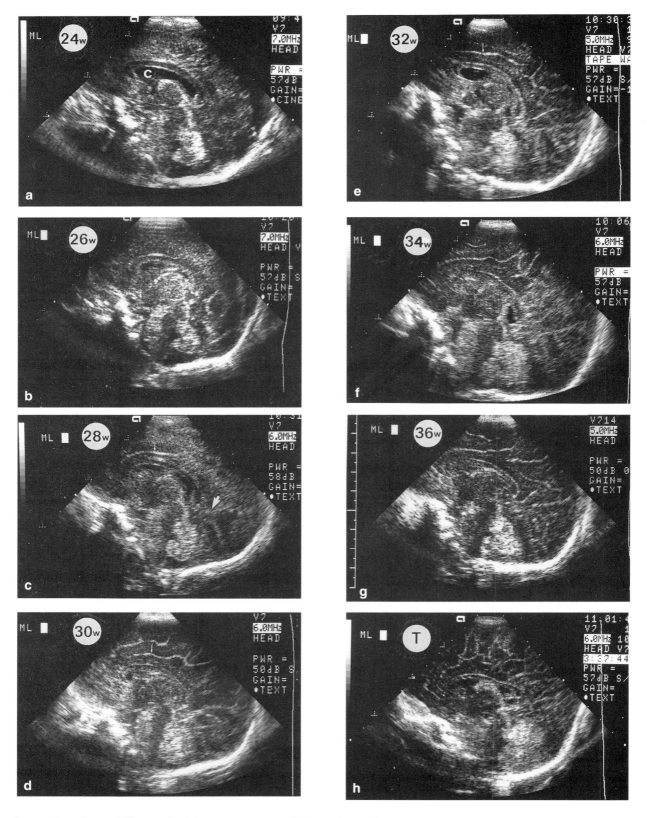

**Figure 15 (a–h)**   Midline sagittal images at two week intervals. With progressive gestation, note the development of the cingulate gyrus and sulci (small arrow) with secondary and tertiary branching. The parieto-occipital fissure (arrow) is also visible as early as 26 weeks gestation and progressively branches. There are many more sulci visible especially after 28 weeks gestation. c, cavum septum pellucidum. Gestation time as indicated on each image (T, term)

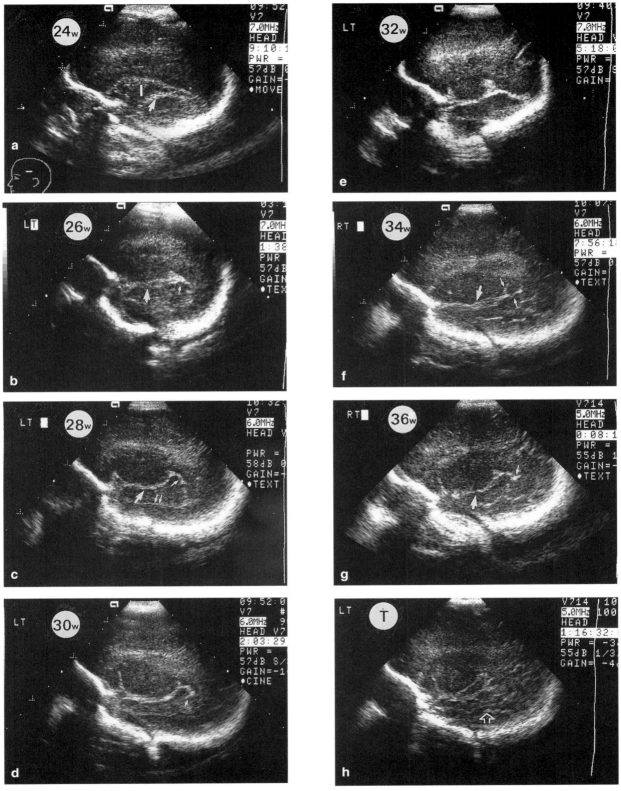

**Figure 16 (a–h)**   Sagittal images through the region of the sylvian fissure at two week intervals. Progressive closure of the exposed insular cortex (I) with formation of the sylvian fissure (large arrow) and secondary and tertiary branching (small arrows) is evident between 24–32 weeks. The superior temporal sulcus (double arrow) and the gyri are easily visible but, at a proper angulation, the inferior temporal sulcus may be visible (open arrow). Gestation time as indicated on each image (T, term)

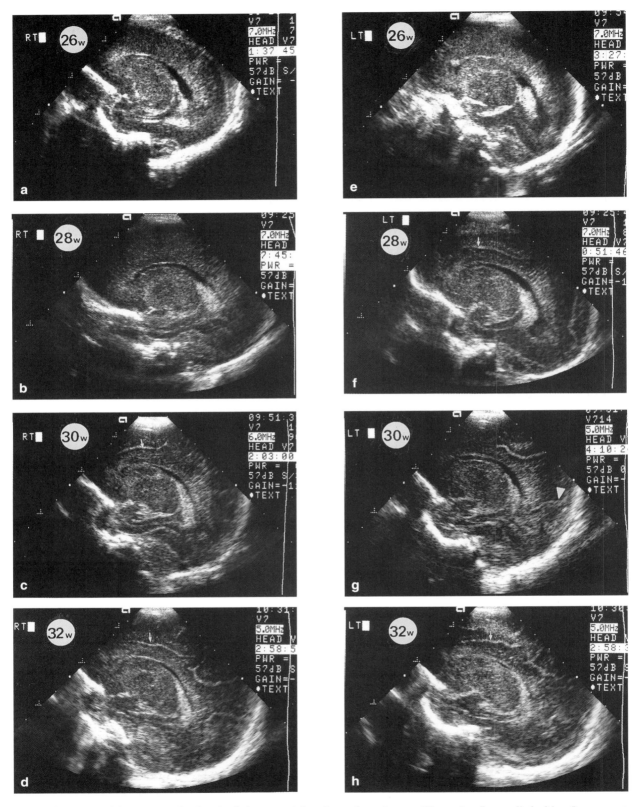

**Figure 17**   Sagittal images at the level of the ventricles show the trigone. There is often a little bit of asymmetry between the right (**a–d**) and the left half (**e–h**) of the brain. Small arrow, cingulate sulci; arrowhead, parieto-occipital fissure. **a & e**, 26 weeks; **b & f**, 28 weeks; **c & g**, 30 weeks; **d & h**, 32 weeks

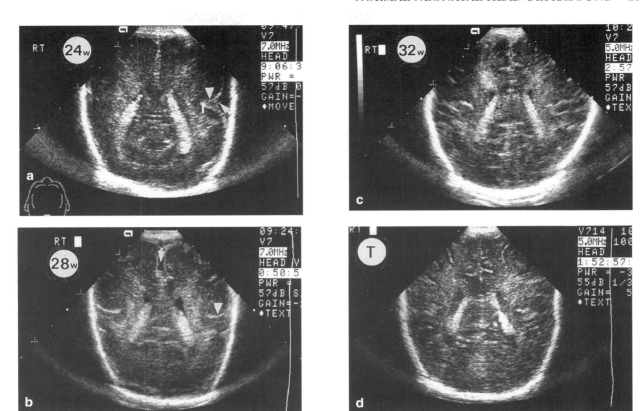

**Figure 18 (a–d)**  Coronal images at the level of the choroid plexus. Note the open sylvian fissure (arrowhead) with exposed insular cortex (I), and the generous subarachnoid fluid (arrow). The brain progressively undergoes sulcation and gyration and the subarachnoid spaces diminish as the brain undergoes maturation. Gestation time as indicated on each image (T, term)

appreciated beyond 26 weeks gestation. It is not a relatively deep sulcus and therefore difficult to visualize and not routinely imaged.

### Parieto-occipital fissure

The parieto-occipital fissure appears at 16 weeks gestation, separating the parietal lobe from the occipital lobe. It begins dorso-medially as the prominent sulcus anatomically and remains fairly distinct until development of secondary sulci in the occipital and parietal lobes[67]. Its presence can be documented on all neonatal head ultrasound beyond 24 weeks[72] (Figures 15 and 17).

### Calcarine fissure

The calcarine fissure appears anatomically by 16 weeks gestation and joins the parieto-occipital fissure anteriorly. The calcarine fissure gradually indents the occipital horn of the lateral ventricle

and appears earlier on the right than on the left side in most cases[67]. On ultrasound, the majority of fetuses will demonstrate the presence of a calcarine fissure by 24–25 weeks and it is seen in 100% beyond 26–27 weeks gestation[72]. It appears as a 'Y' shaped structure and is easily visible.

### Superior, middle and inferior temporal sulci

The superior temporal sulcus appears at 23 weeks gestation, the middle temporal sulcus at 26 weeks gestation, and the inferior temporal sulcus by 30 weeks gestation[67]. However, due to their location along the lateral aspect of the temporal lobe, these are not visible sonographically until these sulci become fairly deep. The inferior temporal sulcus is visible in a minority of individuals by 28–29 weeks gestation and it is the sulcus seen inferior to the sylvian fissure (Figure 16). In the majority of individuals it is visualized by 30–31 weeks gestation and its presence may serve as a clue to gestational age.

*Rolandic (central) and postrolandic (postcentral) sulci*

The rolandic and postrolandic sulci of the parietal lobe appear at 20 and 25 weeks gestation respectively. The rolandic sulcus is a distinct groove in the parasagittal location extending laterally and downwards over the convexity (Figures 11 and 12). The right side may precede the left by as much as 3 weeks. The deep fissure of the central sulcus is evident at 22–23 weeks. Again, due to its location, it is only visible on ultrasound when it is fairly deep. The postrolandic sulcus is visible in approximately 42% of premature neonates at 26–27 weeks gestation and in all neonates by 28–29 weeks gestation[72] (Table 3).

*Periventricular blush*

Nearly all premature newborn infants show increased echogenicity in the periventricular region especially in the peritrigonal regions[56,57] (Figure 18). Its presence is a marker of prematurity. This is demonstrated best on coronal scans through the anterior fontanelles. Its echogenicity does not exceed that of choroid plexus and is homogenous, fine, and symmetrical[56,59]. Hypoechoic CSF separates it from the choroid plexus. Its borders are irregular and poorly defined and the increased echogenicity may not be reproducible when scanning the same region through other 'windows', i.e. posterior fontanelle. This increased periventricular echogenicity is referred to as periventricular blush or halo and, without any complicating factors, disappears with increasing maturity.

*Effaced lateral ventricle*

The isolated finding of the effaced lateral ventricle seen in premature infants (< 36 weeks) is a common finding, occurring in up to 28% of infants[58]. Without accompanying clinical signs of any neurological deficits, the isolated lateral ventricular effacement is not necessarily indicative of hypoxic–ischemic encephalopathy and by itself is not a significant finding[58]. In the term infant, the finding of compressed lateral ventricles or asymmetric lateral ventricles is usually also a normal finding when a parenchymal hemorrhage is excluded and there is no abnormality of the periventricular white matter[59].

## The mature brain

The indications for performing head ultrasound in a term or mature infant are found in Table 1[2,61]. The technique has already been reviewed previously and applies similarly to the mature infant.

*Superficial midline structures*

All the major structures that are visualized when performing head ultrasound will be reviewed (Figure 19). The most superior structure, the superior sagittal sinus, is seen immediately under the anterior fontanelle. In the coronal plane, the superior sagittal sinus is a triangular-shaped structure with hyperechoic boundaries and hypoechoic lumen. Color Doppler is necessary to visualize it (Figure 9). From the apex of this triangular structure is the falx and this is visualized when fluid surrounds it. The surface of the brain is covered with pulsating vessels and these together with the leptomeninges appear as hyperechoic structures. This is easily appreciated when fluid surrounds its convexity. The sulci are deep extensions of the surface and indicate where the pia as well as the vessels have burrowed into the brain and together also appear as hyperechoic structures. The cerebral gyrus consists of both white and gray matter. The gray matter is hypoechoic compared with the white matter which is slightly echogenic. There are medullary vessels within the core of the white matter not found in the gray matter and this probably explains the cause of the hyperechoic central echoes seen within the white matter[73].

*Sulci, fissures and cisterns*

The sulci and the fissures have a variable echogenicity depending on number and size of surface vessels and their width. These, when narrow without any CSF in them, appear hyperechoic and when surrounded by CSF may appear focally or diffusely hypoechoic. Cisterns are CSF spaces surrounding various CNS structures and through which various blood vessels and cranial nerves traverse. Although they contain CSF, they may appear echogenic because of the pulsations, etc., of its contents. The basal cistern (suprasellar cistern) (BC, Figure 19) is visualized in the coronal plane as a crown-shaped cistern which is three-pointed. The midpoint directs upwards towards the interhemispheric fissure and the two lateral points aim towards the cistern of the insulae. It is above the sella and the cavernous sinus lies inferior and lateral to it.

## Midline gyrus and sulci

In the coronal plane, the cingulate sulcus marks the superficial surface of the cingulate gyrus. The interhemispheric fissure often is slightly separated at the level of the cingulate sulcus. Below the margin of the cingulate gyrus is the callosal sulcus which is a horizontal interface perpendicular to the interhemispheric fissure and separates the corpus callosum from the cingulate gyrus. Further inferiorly and anteriorly is the olfactory sulcus, which consists of two obliquely oriented structures that lie to each side of the midline. The gyrus rectus lies between the interhemispheric fissure and the olfactory sulcus on each side. The olfactory gyrus lies just lateral to it. These two gyri are not routinely observed.

## Corpus callosum

The corpus callosum is a thin, sonolucent structure consisting of homogeneously packed bundles of axons crossing the midline just deep to the callosal sulcus and above the cavum septi pellucidi. The corpus callosum consists of rostum, genu, body, and splenium and with the exception of the rostrum develops from anterior to posterior. The genu is visualized between the frontal horns on the coronal scan. In the sagittal plane, the genu, body, and the splenium are identified (Figure 19g).

## Cavum septum pellucidum

The cavum is a trapezoid CSF-containing space located deep to the corpus callosum between the right and the left leaves of the septum pellucidum. Septal veins in it appear as peripheral hyperechoic dots or lines; these are invariably seen in premature infants and less commonly in term infants. Color Doppler demonstrates blood flow in these septal veins.

## Lateral ventricles

The lateral ventricles are divided into five portions: (a) the frontal or anterior horns lie in the frontal lobes anterior to the foramen of Monro.

The frontal horns do not contain choroid plexus and appear as hypoechoic 'wings' that lie immediately lateral to the cavum septum pellucidum. (b) The bodies of the lateral ventricle lie above the third ventricle and thalami and arbitrarily extend from the region of the foramen of Monro anteriorly and the posterior-most portion of the thalamus (pulvinar) posteriorly. The choroid plexus lies along the floor of the ventricles. (c) The atria or the trigone of the lateral ventricles are the widest portion of the ventricles located just posterior to the thalami. The atria are at the confluence of the body, occipital, and temporal horns and contain the glomus of the choroid plexus. (d) The occipital horns of the lateral ventricle extend posteriorly into the occipital lobe. Their size is variable and frequently the occipital horns are asymmetric. The medial aspect of an occipital horn may be indented by a deep calcarine fissure which appears as an ependyma-covered mound and is designated the calcar avis. The occipital horn contains no choroid plexus but occasionally a pedunculated portion of the glomus of the choroid plexus may hang into the occipital horn bilaterally or unilaterally and thus give it a bulky and asymmetrical appearance. (e) The temporal horns extend from the trigone of the lateral ventricle and pass anteriorly and inferiorly into each temporal lobe. They are bounded inferomedially by the hippocampal formation and laterally by the white matter of the temporal lobe. They contain choroid plexus along their entire length.

## Periventricular vasculature

There is prominent periventricular vasculature and these give hypoechoic flares that are best seen in the coronal plane superolateral from the lateral angles of the frontal horn. The major cerebral vasculature, of which the middle cerebral artery is most notable, appear as horizontal tubes with echogenic walls and hypoechoic lumen crossing laterally towards the cistern of the insula on each side in the coronal plane.

## Deep gray nuclei

The deep gray nuclei are a series of large masses of gray matter which lie deep in the brain. The major nuclei are the caudate nucleus, the putamen, the globus pallidus, and the thalamus on each side. The lentiform nucleus or lenticular nucleus is

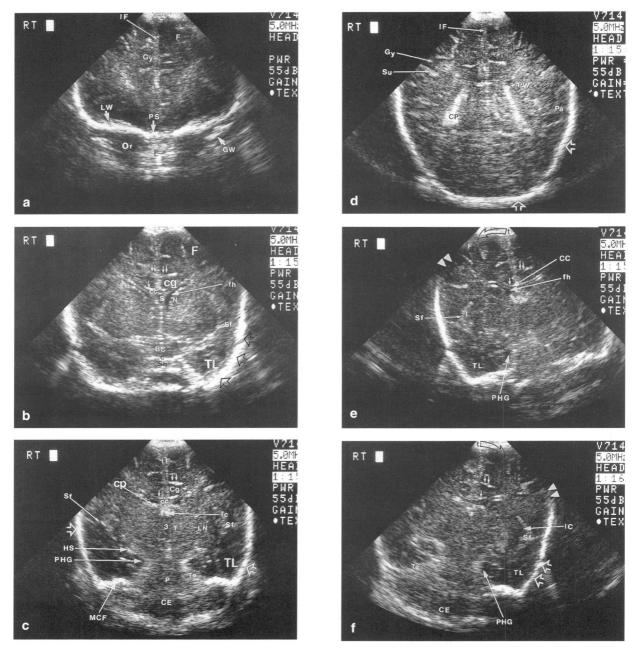

**Figure 19** The mature brain. **a–f**, coronal sector scans; **g–k**, sagittal sector scans; **l**, linear coronal midline images; **m–n**, sagittal linear images. Key to the anatomy: 3rd, 3rd ventricle; 4th, 4th ventricle; AS, aqueduct of sylvius; BC, basal cisterns; C, clivus; CC/cc, corpus callosum; CC-b, body of corpus callosum; CC-g, genu of corpus callosum; CC-s, splenium of corpus callosum; CE, cerebellum; CE-V, cerebellar vermis; Cg, cingulate gyrus; CM, cisterna magna; CP, choroid plexus; CP-g, choroid plexus–glomus; CS/cs, cingulate sulcus on midline sagittal; E, ethmoid complex; F, frontal lobe; fh, frontal horn of lateral ventricle; G, caudothalamic groove; GW, greater wing of sphenoid bone; Gy, gyrus; I, insula; IC, insular cortex; IF, interhemispheric fissure; LF, lateral fissure; LF-a, anterior ascending limb of lateral fissure; LN, lentiform nucleus; LW, lesser wing of sphenoid bone, part of the orbital roof; M, midbrain; MO, medulla oblongata; N, caudate nucleus; O, occipital lobe; OH, occipital horn; Or, orbit; P, pons; Pa, parietal lobe; PHG, parahippocampal gyrus; POF, parieto-occipital fissure; PS, planum sphenoidale; PVE, periventricular echogenicity; PW, periventricular white matter; Q, quadrigeminal plate; S, septum pellucidum; SE–LV, specular echo from roof of lateral ventricle; SF/sf, sylvian fissure; Sh, sphenoid bone; Su, sulcus; T, thalamus; Tc, tela choroidea of 3rd ventricular roof; Te, tentorium cerebelli; TH, temporal horn; TL, temporal lobe; V, vermis of the cerebellum; long black arrow, bony landmark on US; small double arrows, cingulate sulcus on coronal scans; arrowhead, EAF; angled arrow, angled transducer; single white arrow, callosal sulcus.
*Continued on pages 25 and 26*

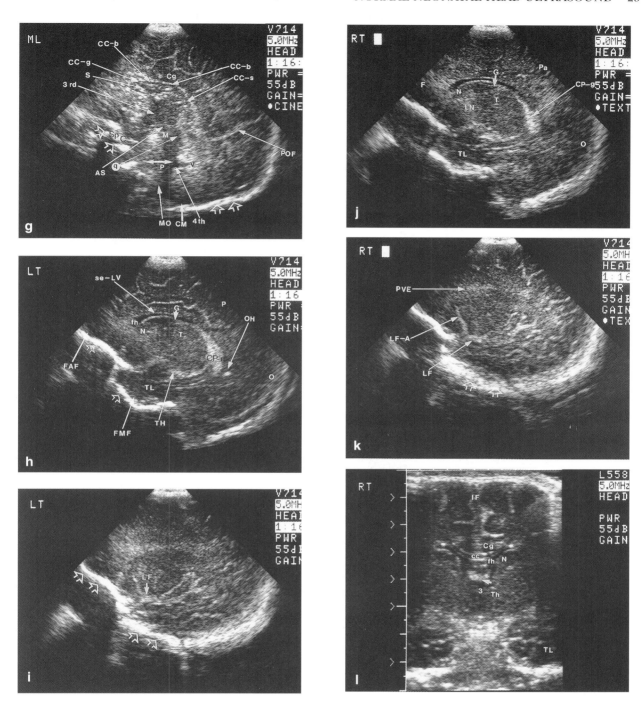

**Figure 19** *Continued*

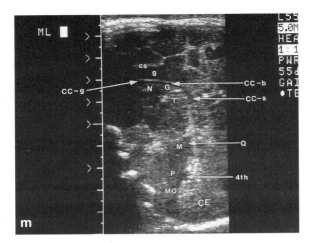

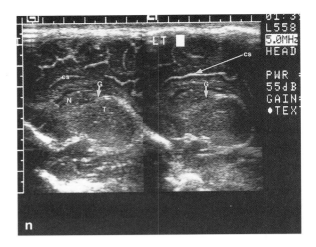

**Figure 19** *Continued*

simply the name given to the globus pallidus plus the putamen nuclei and are so named as together they form a lens-shaped structure. The corpus striatum refers to the combination of the caudate and the putamen nuclei. The name is given because in these deep gray matter pass multiple white fiber bundles of the internal capsule, creating a striated appearance.

## Germinal matrix

The germinal matrix is located in the subependymal region of the frontal horn on the caudate nuclei. It is present prior to 32 weeks gestation and is where subependymal hemorrhage occurs in premature infants.

## Internal capsule

The internal capsule consists of compact bundles of fibers through which all the neural traffic to and from the cerebral cortex passes. These include fibers to the thalamus (cortical thalami fibers), pons via the cerebral peduncle (cortical pontine fibers), motor nuclei of the cranial nerves (cortical bulbar fibers), spinal cord motor neurons (cortical spinal fibers), and also to other regions of the cerebral cortex and basal ganglia (corticocortical fibers). This structure is not routinely appreciated on ultrasound.

## Choroid plexus

The ventricular system is roofed by a layer of ependymal cells overlaid by a layer of pia. The pia in all other locations faces the subarachnoid space and is where the blood vessels are located. This pia–ependyma complex in certain locations invaginates into the ventricles forming a collection of arterials, venules, and capillaries covered by secondary cuboidal epithelium (choroidal epithelium). This entire ependyma–pia–capillary complex is the choroid plexus. It is absent in the frontal/anterior horn and the occipital/posterior horns of the lateral ventricle and is absent in the aqueduct. In all remaining areas of the ventricular system, it is found. It is seen coursing through the body of the lateral ventricle to the interventricular foramen. In the atria, it is called the glomus (Latin for ball of thread). It is also found in the roof of the third ventricle as well as the caudal half of the fourth ventricle.

## Insula, circular sulcus and operculum

The gray matter forming the surface of the brain that is lateral to the external capsule is the insula. It is relatively hyperechoic and is surrounded superiorly and inferiorly by the circular sulcus. It is an area of cerebral cortex not included in any of the four lobes that lie buried in the depth of the lateral sulcus. The insula overlies the site where the telencephalon and the diencephalon fuse during embryological development. The operculum is the portion of a given lobe of a cerebral cortex overlying the insula and thus concealing it from anatomical visualization; there is frontal, parietal, or temporal operculum.

## Extra-axial fluid

Fluid in the extra-axial space (subdural and subarachnoid) is easily detected by ultrasound and is frequently seen in normal babies, both premature and mature[33–35,74–77]. It can be noted in the interhemispheric fissure and over the convexities (Figure 14 at 24 weeks).

Since extra-axial fluid can occur, its presence must be correlated with the infant's clinical condition and neurological status.

## Summary

In this chapter, we have briefly reviewed the relevant embryology and the technique of performing a standard neonatal head ultrasound. The bony landmarks and key anatomical structures viewed have been discussed. The attention paid to these details while performing and acquiring head ultrasound images makes one study easily comparable with another. The vascular anatomy of the brain, referring to major vessels, was reviewed and their observance on color and power Doppler was included. The key structures in the changing brain were reviewed sequentially to appreciate evolving maturity. The mature brain, the key anatomical structures, and labeled ultrasound images conclude this chapter. This background provides a working foundation to proceed to the next chapters.

## Acknowledgments

We would like to thank all the US technologists: Tracy Johnston, Audrey Touchette, Joni Levine, Debbie Stamplis, Hina Shah, and especially Donna Schave and Sally Thompson, for the technical care in acquiring the images depicted in this chapter. We appreciate the audiovisual department, especially Cliff Roberts who reproduced the numerous images, and all the help from Michele Klein and her library staff. We would also like to thank Dr Larry Kuhns for his assistance and Jennifer Handley for typing and preparing the manuscript.

# References

1. Leksell L. Echoencephalography: detection of the intracranial complications following head injury. *Acta Chir Scand* 1956;110:301–15

2. Slovis TL. Real-time ultrasound of the intracranial contents. In Haller JO, Shkolnik A, eds. *Ultrasound in Pediatrics*. New York: Churchill Livingstone, 1981,13–27

3. Kossoff G, Garrett WJ, Radavanovic G. Ultrasonic atlas of normal brain of infant. *Ultrasound Med Biol* 1974;1:259–66

4. Garrett WJ, Kossoff G, Jones RHC. Ultrasonic cross-sectional visualization of hydrocephalus in infants. *Neuroradiology* 1975;8:279–88

5. Yousefzadeh DK, Naidich TP. US anatomy of the posterior fossa in children: correlation with brain sections. *Radiology* 1985;156:353–61

6. Naidich TP, Yousefzadeh DK, Gusnard DA. Sonography of the normal neonatal head. *Neuroradiology* 1986;28:408–27

7. Goldstein RB, Filly RA, Toi A. Septal veins: a normal finding on neonatal cranial sonography. *Radiology* 1986;161:623–4

8. Naidich TP, Gusnard DA, Yousefzadeh DK. Sonography of the internal capsule and basal ganglia in infants: 1. Coronal sections. *Am J Neuroradiol* 1985;6:909–17

9. Pigadas A, Thompson JR, Grube GL. Normal infant brain anatomy: correlated real-time sonograms and brain specimens. *Am J Roent* 1981;137:815–20

10. Shuman WP, Rogers JV, Mack LA, *et al*. Real-time sonographic sector scanning of the neonatal cranium: technique and normal anatomy. *Am J Roent* 1981;137:821–8

11. Fiske CE, Filly RA, Callen PW. The normal choroid plexus: ultrasonographic appearance of the neonatal head. *Radiology* 1981;141:467–71

12. Rosenberg HK, Stoltz KA. A new technique to visualize the convexities of the brain using real-time ultrasound. *J Clin Ultrasound* 1983;11:56–8

13. Cremin BJ, Chilton SJ, Peacock WJ. Anatomical landmarks in anterior fontanelle ultrasonography. *Br J Radiol* 1983;56:517–26

14. Poland RL, Slovis TL, Shankaran S. Normal values for ventricular size as determined by real time sonographic techniques. *Pediatr Radiol* 1985;15:12–14

15. Perry RNW, Bowman ED, Roy RND, *et al*. Ventricular size in newborn infants. *J Ultrasound Med* 1985;4:475–7

16. Johnson ML, Mack LA, Rumack CM, *et al*. B-mode echoencephalography in the normal and high risk infant. *Am J Radiol* 1979;133:375–81

17. Haber K, Wachter RD, Christenson PC, *et al*. Ultrasonic evaluation of intracranial pathology in infants: a new technique. *Radiology* 1980;134:173–8

18. Babcock DS, Han BK, LeQuesne GW. B-mode gray scale ultrasound of the head in the newborn and young infant. *Am J Radiol* 1980;134:457–68

19. Slovis TL, Kuhns LR. Real-time sonography of the brain through the anterior fontanelle. *Am J Radiol* 1981;136:277–86

20. Sauerbrei EE, Harrison PB, Ling E, *et al.* Neonatal intracranial pathology demonstrated by high-frequency linear array ultrasound. *J Clin Ultrasound* 1981;9:33–6

21. Edwards MK, Brown DL, Muller J, *et al.* Cribside neurosonography: real-time sonography for intracranial investigation of the neonate. *Am J Radiol* 1981;136:271–6

22. Babcock DS, Han BK. The accuracy of high resolution, real-time ultrasonography of the head in infancy. *Radiology* 1981;139:665–76

23. Grant EG, Schellinger D, Borts FT, *et al.* Real-time sonography of the neonatal and infant head. *Am J Radiol* 1981;136:265–70

24. Volpe JJ. Editor's column. Anterior fontanel: window to the neonatal brain. *J Pediatr* 1982;100:395–8

25. Siegel MJ, Patel J, Gado MH, *et al.* Cranial computed tomography and real-time sonography in full-term neonates and infants. *Radiology* 1983;149: 111–16

26. Naidich TP, Yousefzadeh DK, Gusnard DA, *et al.* Sonography of the internal capsule and basal ganglia in infants. Part II. Localization of pathological processes in sagittal section through the caudothalamic groove. *Radiology* 1986;161:615–21

27. Slovis TL, Canady A, Touchette A, *et al.* Transcranial sonography through the burr hole for detection of ventriculomegaly. *J Ultrasound Med* 1991;10:195–200

28. Cohen HL, Haller JO. Advances in perinatal neurosonography. *Am J Radiol* 1994;163:801–10

29. Babcock DS. Sonography of the brain in infants: role in evaluating neurologic abnormalities. *Am J Radiol* 1995;165:417–23

30. Grant EG, Schellinger D, Richardson JD. Real-time ultrasonography of the posterior fossa. *J Ultrasound Med* 1983;2:73–87

31. Winchester P, Brill PW, Cooper R, *et al.* Prevalence of 'compressed' and asymmetric lateral ventricles in healthy full-term neonates: sonographic study. *Am J Roent* 1986;146:471–5

32. Patel MD, Cheng AG, Callen PW. Lateral ventricular effacement as an isolated sonographic finding in premature infants: prevalence and significance. *Am J Radiol* 1995;165:155–9

33. Grant EG, Jacobs NM. Sonographic appearance of extra-axial fluid collections in the infant: further observations. *J Clin Ultrasound* 1984;12:339–42

34. Kleinman PK, Zito JL, Davidson RI, *et al.* The subarachnoid spaces in children: normal variations in size. *Radiology* 1983;147:455–7

35. Ment LR, Duncan CC, Geehr R. Benign enlargement of the subarachnoid space in the infant. *J Neurosurg* 1981;54:504–8

36. Robertson WC Jr, Chun RWM, Orrison WW, *et al.* Benign subdural collections of infancy. *J Pediatr* 1979;94:382–5

37. Fischer AQ, Aziz E. Diagnosis of cerebral atrophy in infants by near-field cranial sonography. *Am J Dis Child* 1986;140:774–7

38. Grant EG, Schellinger D, Richardson JD, *et al.* Echogenic periventricular halo: normal sonographic finding or neonatal cerebral hemorrhage. *Am J Radiol* 1983;140:793–6

39. DiPietro MA, Brody BA, Teele RL. Peritrigonal echogenic 'blush' on cranial sonography: pathological correlates. *Am J Radiol* 1986;146:1067–72

40. Fakhry J, Schechter A, Tenner MS, *et al.* Cysts of the choroid plexus in neonates: documentation and review of the literature. *J Ultrasound Med* 1985;4: 561–3

41. Goodwin L, Quisling RG. The neonatal cisterna magna: ultrasonic evaluation. *Radiology* 1983;149: 691–5

42. Bowie JD, Kirks DR, Rosenberg ER, *et al.* Caudothalamic groove: value in identification of germinal matrix hemorrhage by sonography in preterm neonates. *Am J Neuroradiol* 1983;4:1107–10

43. DiPietro MA, Brody BA, Teele RL. The calcar avis: demonstration with cranial US. *Radiology* 1985;156: 363–4

44. Mitchell DG, Merton DA, Mirsky PJ, *et al.* Circle of Willis in newborns: color Doppler imaging of 53 healthy full-term infants. *Radiology* 1989;172:201–5

45. Mitchell DG, Merton D, Needleman L, *et al.* Neonatal brain: color Doppler imaging, part 1. Technique and vascular anatomy. *Radiology* 1988;167:303–6

46. Bezinque SL, Slovis TL, Touchette AS, *et al.* Characterization of superior sagittal sinus blood flow velocity using color flow Doppler in neonates and infants. *Pediatr Radiol* 1995;25:175–9

47. Segal SR, Rosenberg HK. Sonographic appearance of the torcular herophili. *Am J Radiol* 1986;146: 109–12

48. Dean LM, Taylor GA. The intracranial venous system in infants: normal and abnormal findings on duplex and color Doppler sonography. *Am J Radiol* 1995;164:151–6

49. Lupetin AR, Davis DA, Beckman I, *et al.* Transcranial Doppler sonography. Part 1. Principles, technique, and normal appearances. *RadioGraphics* 1995;15:179–91

50. Lupetin AR, Davis DA, Beckman I, *et al.* Transcranial Doppler sonography. Part 2. Evaluation of intracranial and extracranial abnormalities and procedural monitoring. *RadioGraphics* 1995;15: 193–209

51. Luker GD, Siegel MJ. Sinus pericranii: sonographic findings. *Am J Radiol* 1995;165:175–6

52. Wang H-S, Kuo M-F. Supraorbital approach of the anterior cerebral artery: a new window for transcranial Doppler sonography. *J Ultrasound Med* 1995;14:259–61

53. Cubberley DA, Jaffe RB, Nixon GW. Sonographic demonstration of Galenic arteriovenous malformations in the neonate. *Am J Neuroradiol* 1982;3: 435–9

54. Soto G, Daneman A, Hellman J. Doppler evaluation of cerebral arteries in a Galenic vein malformation. *J Ultrasound Med* 1985;4:673–5

55. Williams JL. Intracranial vascular pulsations in pediatric neurosonology. *J Ultrasound Med* 1983;2:485–8

56. Moore KL. *The Developing Human: Clinically Oriented Embryology*, 4th edn. Philadelphia: W.B. Saunders, 1988:364–401

57. Kostović I, Judaš M. Prenatal development of the cerebral cortex. In Chervenek FA, Kurjak A, Comstock CH, eds. *Ultrasound and the Fetal Brain*. New York: Parthenon Publishing, 1995;1–26

58. Hansen PE, Ballesteros MC, Soila K, *et al*. MR imaging of the developing human brain. *RadioGraphics* 1993;13:21–36

59. Ballesteros MC, Hansen PE, Soila K. MR imaging of the developing human brain. Part 2: Postnatal development. *RadioGraphics* 1993;13:611–22

60. Sudakoff G, Montazemi M, Riflin M. The foramen magnum: the underutilized acoustic window to the posterior fossa. *J Ultrasound Med* 1993;4:205–10

61. Sims ME, Halterman G, Jasani N, *et al*. Indications for routine cranial ultrasound scanning in the nursery. *J Clin Ultrasound* 1986;14:443–7

62. DiPietro MA, Faix RG, Donn SM. Procedural hazards of neonatal ultrasonography. *J Clin Ultrasound* 1986;14:361–6

63. Cahill DR. Parasagittal anatomy of the head and neck. *Mayo Clin Proc* 1986;61:127–39

64. deGroot J. *Correlative Neuroanatomy*, 21st edn. Norwalk, Connecticut: Appleton & Lange, 1991:129–31

65. Turner OA. Growth and development of the cerebral cortical pattern in man. *Arch Neurol Psych* 1948;59:1–12

66. Dorovini-Zis K, Dolman CL. Gestational development of brain. *Arch Pathol Lab Med* 1977;101:192–5

67. Chi JG, Dooling EC, Gilles FH. Gyral development of the human brain. *Ann Neurol* 1977;1:86–93

68. Scher MS, Barmada MA. Estimation of gestational age by electrographic, clinical, and anatomic criteria. *Pediatr Neurol* 1987;3:256–62

69. Worthen NJ, Gilbertson V, Lau C. Cortical sulcal development seen on sonography: relationship to gestational parameters. *J Ultrasound Med* 1986;5:153–6

70. Slagle TA, Oliphant M, Gross SJ. Cingulate sulcus development in preterm infants. *Pediatr Res* 1989;26:598–602

71. Murphy NP, Rennie J, Cooke RWI. Cranial ultrasound assessment of gestational age in low birthweight infants. *Arch Dis Child* 1989;64:569–72

72. Huang CC. Sonographic cerebral sulcal development in premature newborns. *Brain Dev* 1991;13:27–31

73. Naidich TP, Grant JL, Altman N, *et al*. The developing cerebral surface. *Neuroimag Clin North Am* 1994;4:201–39

74. Slovis TL, Kelly JK, Eisenbrey AB, *et al*. Detection of extracerebral fluid collections by real-time sector scanning through the anterior fontanelle. *J Ultrasound Med* 1982;1:41–4

75. Babcock DS, Han BK, Dine MS. Sonographic findings in infants with macrocrania. *Am J Radiol* 1988;150:1359–65

76. Prassopoulos P, Cavouras D, Goldinopoulos S, *et al*. The size of the intra- and extraventricular cerebrospinal fluid compartments in children with idiopathic benign widening of the frontal subarachnoid space. *Neuroradiology* 1995;37:418–21

77. Hamza M, Bodensteiner JB, Noorani PA, *et al*. Benign extracerebral fluid collections: a cause of macrocrania in infancy. *Pediatr Neurol* 1987;3:218–21

# Neonatal sonography: congenital malformations of the brain

## 2

*Megan K. Dishop, Sam T. Auringer and Thomas E. Sumner*

---

Ultrasound has become an important method for the detection of congenital brain malformations in neonates. Although it does not possess the contrast and spatial resolution capabilities of computed tomography (CT) or magnetic resonance imaging (MRI), ultrasound has nevertheless proven highly effective for the diagnosis of major structural malformations and is the preferred screening study for neonates suspected of having a brain malformation[1–4]. For example, malformation should be suspected in any infant with an enlarged head, craniofacial dysmorphism, a chromosomal anomaly such as trisomy 13–15 or 18, spinal dysraphism, myelomeningocele, unexplained seizures, or abnormal neurologic findings[2,3,5,6]. In such cases, sonography through the anterior fontanelle is an ideal initial study of intracranial anatomy.

Ultrasound is well-suited for the very young patient because it is a safe and rapid neuroimaging study that requires neither sedation nor radiation. It is practical within the neonatal intensive care environment as its portability allows imaging at the cribside. The real-time multiplanar and Doppler capabilities of ultrasound, its relatively low cost, and the inherent sonographic contrast between brain and cerebrospinal fluid (CSF) make ultrasound an attractive modality for use in neonatal neuroimaging[1,3,7–10].

This chapter highlights the common congenital brain malformations detectable by sonography. The sonographic appearance of normal structures is first presented, followed by a discussion of the embryologic classification of congenital brain malformations. Each malformation is then described in terms of gross pathology, etiology and pathogenesis if known, associated anomalies, and clinical manifestations. Emphasis is placed on describing the key sonographic findings that allow diagnosis and differentiation of the major congenital brain malformations. In addition to sonographic images, other forms of neuroimaging have been included to clarify the anatomy of each malformation and to emphasize the role of integrated neuroimaging.

## Normal anatomy

The sonographic diagnosis of congenital brain malformations requires a working knowledge of the normal midline and ventricular anatomy of the neonatal brain, as most of the common congenital malformations disrupt the midline anatomy and may cause dilatation of the ventricles due to associated hydrocephalus (Figure 1).

## Embryology and classification

Normal development of the brain is an extraordinarily complex process which is prone to a wide variety of insults, both genetic and environmental[1]. Van der Knaap & Valk[11] classify congenital malformations of the brain into categories based on the stage of development at which the abnormality occurs. Four major categories may be identified: (1) disorders of dorsal induction; (2) disorders of ventral induction; (3) disorders of histogenesis, proliferation, and differentiation; and (4) disorders of migration.

Normal development begins with the process of dorsal induction which refers to formation of the neural tube, the precursor to the brain and spinal cord. Dorsal induction can be divided into (1) primary neurulation, i.e. formation of the neural tube in the cranial direction from the level of L1–L2, and (2) secondary neurulation, i.e. formation of the caudal neural tube. The next stage is ventral induction, which refers to the development of the rostral embryo to form the face, optic vesicles, and brain. This process involves division of the primitive brain into the prosencephalon, mesencephalon, and rhombencephalon, which will eventually become the mature cerebral hemispheres, cerebellum, and brainstem. After the general form of the brain is established, a number of processes occur simultaneously which allow for the specialization and complexity of the mature brain. These processes include histogenesis, proliferation, and differentiation. Histogenesis is

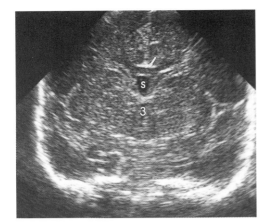

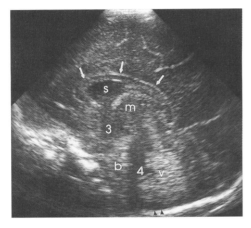

**Figure 1** Normal anatomy. Coronal (**a**) and sagittal (**b**) midline images reveal the brainstem (b), cerebellar vermis (v), cisterna magna (arrowheads), corpus callosum (arrows), massa intermedia (m), cavum septum pellucidum (s), and the lateral, third (3), and fourth (4) ventricles

the development of cells into tissues, for example as occurs in the formation of blood vessels. Proliferation is an increase in the number of cells, while differentiation is an increase in the types of cells. The last stage involves migration of the primitive neuroblasts from the periventricular region to the cortex, causing formation of gyri and sulci. Formation of the major interhemispheric commisures such as the corpus callosum is associated with this neuronal migration[11,12].

Because errors may occur at any one of these steps in development, a wide array of different brain malformations have been recognized[13]. The most common malformations diagnosable by cranial sonography will be discussed here using these four developmental stages as a framework (Table 1).

**Table 1** Major congenital brain malformations detectable by sonography (based on van der Knaap and Valk classification[11])

Dorsal induction (3–4 weeks)
    Chiari II malformation
    Encephalocele
Ventral induction (5–10 weeks)
    Dandy–Walker malformation
    Holoprosencephaly
    Septo-optic dysplasia
    Absence of the septum pellucidum
Histogenesis, proliferation, and differentiation (8–20 weeks)
    Vein of Galen malformation
    Hydranencephaly
    Aqueductal stenosis
    Hemimegalencephaly
Migration (8–20 weeks)
    Schizencephaly
    Lissencephaly
    Agenesis of the corpus callosum

## Disorders of dorsal induction

### Chiari II malformation

The Chiari malformations are anomalies of the hindbrain which are associated with hydrocephalus. The Chiari I malformation refers to inferior displacement of the cerebellar tonsils in a triangular shape through a small foramen magnum. The Chiari II malformation is a complex anomaly involving a small posterior fossa and inferior displacement of the cerebellum and brainstem through a large foramen magnum, and is associated with a myelomeningocele. The Chiari III malformation is a rare condition consisting of a low occipital and/or high cervical encephalocele with other features of the Chiari II malformation[12]. Chiari II will be the focus of our discussion as it is the most common Chiari malformation in the neonatal period.

The Chiari II malformation is a hindbrain anomaly in which the inferior cerebellum, tonsils, brainstem, and fourth ventricle are caudally displaced through an enlarged foramen magnum into the cervical spinal canal[12,14,15]. The posterior fossa is small and the tentorium is low-lying with a large incisura[12,16]. Additional findings may include tectal breaking of the midbrain, dorsal kinking of the cervicomedullary junction, and scalloping of the petrous pyramids and clivus[12,16]. Hydrocephalus is common due to obstruction at the level of the foramen magnum[1,7]. The Chiari II malformation is also highly associated with spinal dysraphism, as it is found in 85–90% of myelomeningocele patients[13,15]. Other possible findings include agenesis of the corpus callosum, fenestration of the falx with interdigitation of the medial cortical gyri, aqueductal stenosis, heterotopic gray matter, polymicrogyria, and hydromyelia[16,17].

The Chiari II malformation is thought to be caused by a failure in neural tube formation due to the absence of specific surface molecules, which not only causes a myelomeningocele caudally, but also causes failed expansion of the ventricular system rostrally[18]. The lack of inductive pressure in the forming ventricles results in a small posterior fossa and incomplete separation of the thalami. As the cerebellum and brainstem develop in an abnormally confining posterior fossa, they cause the formation of a dysplastic tentorium and an enlarged foramen magnum, through which they herniate into the spinal canal[18].

## Sonographic findings

Sonographic findings of the Chiari II malformation[1,2,3,7,13–15] (Figures 2 and 3) include:

(1)  A small posterior fossa with caudal displacement of the hindbrain.
(2)  Poor visualization and elongation of the fourth ventricle. If apparent, the fourth ventricle is low relative to the occipital bone, and in severe cases may be outside of the skull.
(3)  Obliteration of the cisterna magna.
(4)  A large massa intermedia (interthalamic adhesion), which may obscure the third ventricle in part.
(5)  Dilatation of the lateral ventricles due to hydrocephalus, often asymmetrically. The ventricles may occasionally be of normal size.
(6)  Superior squaring and inferior pointing of the frontal horns, giving them a 'bat wing' appearance in the coronal plane.
(7)  Colpocephaly. This refers to a fetal configuration of the ventricles in which the occipital horns and atria of the lateral ventricles are larger than the frontal or temporal horns, with the cerebral mantle thinnest over the occipital horns.
(8)  Prominent choroid plexus in the lateral ventricles consisting of an elongated glomus terminating in a club-like nodule (a 'drumstick' configuration).

Other findings of the Chiari II malformation may include a prominent anterior commisure, herniation of the third ventricle into the suprasellar cistern, an enlarged suprapineal recess, a prominent interhemispheric fissure, a hypoplastic falx, and a hypoplastic tentorium with a large incisura[1,7,13].

### Encephalocele

An encephalocele is a dysraphic condition in which intracranial contents including brain tissue herniate through a defect in the skull[3]. Although they show great variability in size and shape, encephaloceles are typically rounded, skin-covered masses which may be either broad based or pedunculated[19]. They occur most commonly in the occipital region, but may also occur in the parietal, ethmoid, sphenoid, nasal, orbital, or frontal regions[2,3]. They may be isolated anomalies or may be associated with the Chiari III malformation, the Dandy–Walker complex, diastematomyelia, or Klippel–Feil syndrome.

## Sonographic findings

Sonographic findings of an encephalocele include[14]:

(1)  An opening in the cranium with the stalk of the encephalocele extending through it (Figure 4).
(2)  A sac which contains displaced intracranial contents, including echogenic neural tissue and ventricles.

Although an encephalocele can be diagnosed on clinical examination, sonography is useful in detecting associated malformations and in determining the amount of brain tissue contained within the sac preoperatively[2,3,13,17].

## Disorders of ventral induction

### Dandy–Walker malformation

The Dandy–Walker malformation (DWM) is a cystic abnormality consisting of an enlarged posterior fossa with a high position of the tentorium, hypoplasia of the cerebellar vermis, and massive dilatation of the fourth ventricle filling the posterior fossa[15,20]. It is a component of the Dandy–Walker complex, a term which encompasses

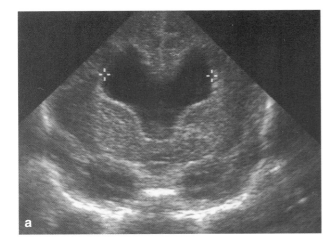

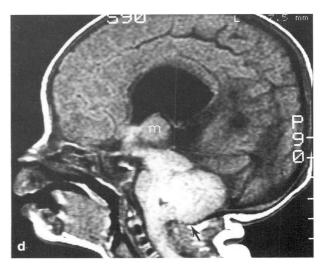

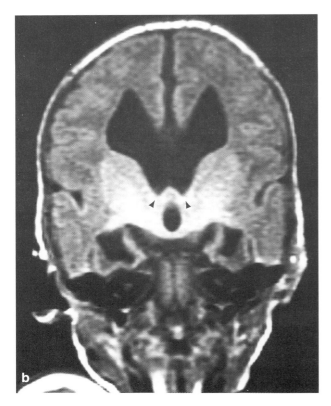

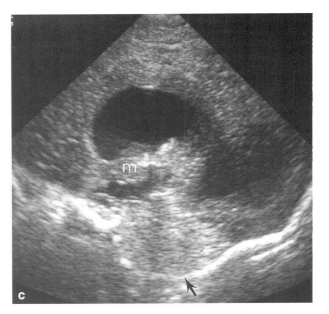

**Figure 2** Chiari II malformation. Coronal US and MR images (**a** and **b**) demonstrate the characteristic superior squaring (+) and inferior pointing (arrowheads) of the dilated frontal horns of the lateral ventricles. Sagittal US and MR images (**c** and **d**) demonstrate the classic small posterior fossa, poor visualization of the elongated fourth ventricle, obliteration of the cisterna magna (arrow), and the large massa intermedia (m)

a continuum of posterior fossa cystic abnormalities, including the Dandy–Walker malformation, the Dandy–Walker variant, and the mega-cisterna magna. All three are thought to be caused by insults to the developing cerebellum and fourth ventricle, but differ in terms of the resulting size of the posterior fossa and the degree of cerebellar hypoplasia[20]. The Dandy–Walker variant consists of hypoplasia of the cerebellar vermis and cystic dilatation of the fourth ventricle, but without enlargement of the posterior fossa as in DWM[20]. A

mega-cisterna magna refers to an enlarged posterior fossa secondary to an enlarged cisterna magna, without a dilated fourth ventricle or cerebellar hypoplasia[20].

The etiology of the DWM remains unclear[21]. It has been attributed to atresia or delayed opening of the foramina of Luschka and Magendie during the fifth to tenth week of gestation, with resultant obstruction of CSF outflow from the fourth

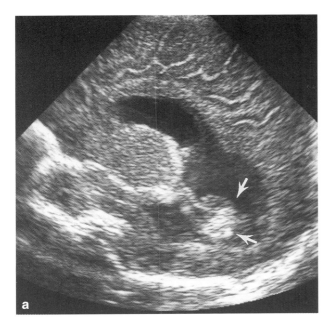

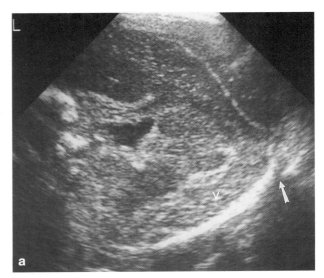

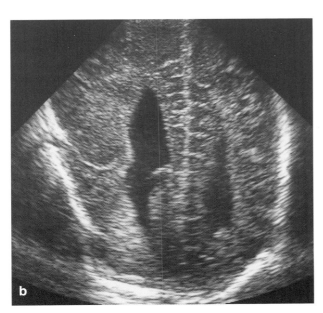

**Figure 3** Chiari II malformation. Sagittal (**a**) and coronal (**b**) images of an infant with myelomeningocele demonstrate the prominent drumstick or nodular configuration of the lateral ventricular choroid plexus (arrows) and asymmetric dilatation of the colpocephalic lateral ventricles

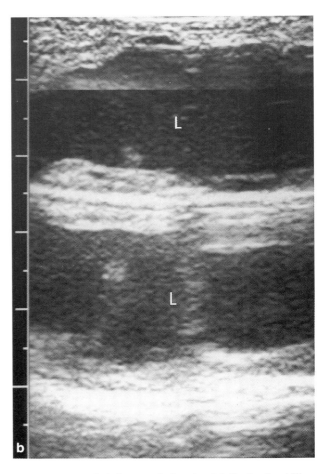

**Figure 4** Occipital encephalocele. (**a**) Sagittal midline image demonstrates a gap in the occipital bone (arrow) through which echogenic neural tissue protrudes. The vermis (v) appears stretched. (**b**) Transverse image of the encephalocele reveals it to contain the dilated lateral ventricles (L)

ventricle[22]. However, other investigators have suggested that the cyst results from some other as yet undetermined source of increased intraventricular pressure[1,2,7,21].

Patients with the Dandy–Walker malformation may present with increased head circumference, postnatal hydrocephalus or developmental delay[15,20–22]. Additional clinical findings may include seizures, hearing or visual difficulty, congenital cardiac abnormalities, and polydactyly[15,23]. Other central nervous system (CNS) abnormalities include agenesis of the corpus callosum, heterotopic gray matter, aqueductal stenosis, occipital encephaloceles, polymicrogyria, cysts in the thalamic–hypothalamic region, and holoprosencephaly[1,7,15,24,25]. Prognosis is variable depending on the severity of the malformation[2].

## Sonographic findings

Sonographic findings of the DWM[1,2,7,13–15,23,26] (Figure 5) include:

(1) An enlarged posterior fossa containing a large fluid-filled anechoic cyst communicating with the fourth ventricle. Although a midline sagittal view usually provides the best view, an axial image through the temporal squama may be helpful in demonstrating the contour of the cyst and its communication with the fourth ventricle.
(2) Partial or complete absence of the cerebellar vermis.
(3) Hypoplasia and anterolateral displacement of the cerebellar hemispheres.
(4) Elevation of the tentorium.
(5) Variable dilatation of the third and lateral ventricles.
(6) Divergence of the occipital horns due to anterolateral displacement.
(7) Obliteration of the basal cisterns.

The DWM should be distinguished sonographically from the other components of the complex. The Dandy–Walker variant typically shows a less hypoplastic vermis and a posterior fossa normal in size, while the mega-cisterna magna shows an intact vermis but with an enlarged posterior fossa[23]. Because these entities represent a continuum, there is no single characteristic which definitively distinguishes them.

The DWM must also be distinguished from a posterior fossa arachnoid cyst. An arachnoid cyst is a collection of CSF due to pial layer entrapment

which may exert a mass effect[1,2,25]. In contrast to the DWM, an arachnoid cyst shows an intact cerebellar vermis and a lack of communication with the fourth ventricle[1,27]. Finally, the DWM should be distinguished from post-hemorrhagic enlargement or trapping of the fourth ventricle, which in contrast develops over time, causes a lesser dilatation of the third and lateral ventricles, and lacks an elevated tentorium[3].

### Holoprosencephaly

Holoprosencephaly is a rare disorder of diverticulation in which the forebrain (prosencephalon) fails to cleave in the midline and develop bilaterally[6]. The prosencephalon is composed of the telencephalon (cerebral hemispheres) and the diencephalon (thalamus and hypothalamus)[15]. As a result, these structures remain fused instead of separating bilaterally. Variable fusion of the olfactory tracts and optic tracts is also seen[15].

Holoprosencephaly is caused by an abnormality of the rostral notochord which occurs in the fourth to the eighth week of gestation[15]. It has many associated causes including trisomy 13-15, trisomy 18, maternal diabetes mellitus, intrauterine rubella, and toxoplasmosis[1,7]. Because the fetal face is developing at the same time, these infants often have associated facial anomalies, such as cyclopia, hypotelorism, cleft lip and palate, micrognathia, absence of the nasal septum, and trigonocephaly[1,7,13,15].

Holoprosencephaly is classified into three subtypes based on degree of diverticulation and therefore severity–alobar, semilobar, and lobar[15].

## Alobar holoprosencephaly

Alobar is the most severe type of holoprosencephaly, characterized by complete absence of diverticulation[12]. If not stillborn, these children have significant hypotonia, apnea, and seizures, and usually die in the neonatal period[28]. Sonographic findings of alobar holoprosencephaly[1–3,7,12,13,15] (Figures 6 and 7) include:

(1) A single large horseshoe-shaped ventricle.
(2) Fused echogenic thalami.
(3) A thin mantle of undifferentiated parenchyma over the monoventricle.
(4) Absence of the interhemispheric fissure and third ventricle.
(5) Agenesis of the corpus callosum.
(6) Normal cerebellum and brainstem.

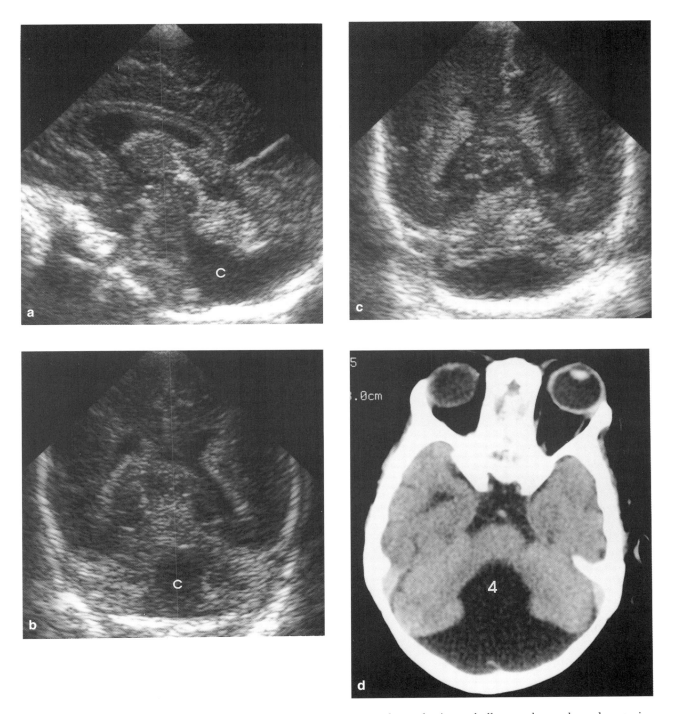

**Figure 5**  Dandy–Walker complex. (**a**) Sagittal view demonstrates a hypoplastic cerebellum and an enlarged posterior fossa which contains a fluid-filled cyst (c) communicating with the fourth ventricle. (**b**) Coronal view shows the fluid collection (c) in the posterior fossa. (**c** and **d**) Coronal view and CT images show absence of the cerebellar vermis, with the CT also demonstrating communication of the posterior fossa fluid with the fourth ventricle (4)

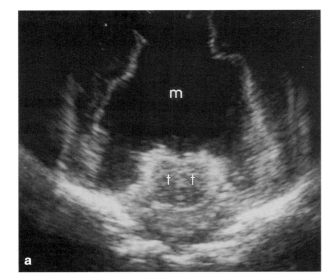

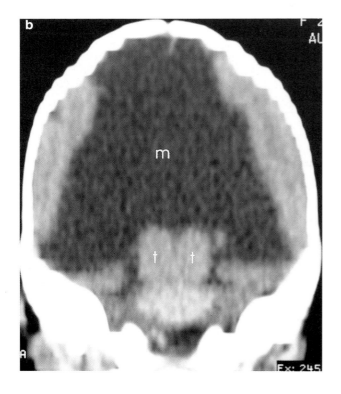

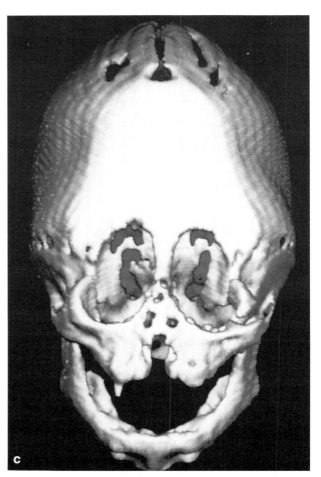

**Figure 6** Alobar holoprosencephaly. Images of an infant with trisomy 13. (**a**) Coronal US and (**b**) reconstructed oblique coronal CT show a large monoventricle (m), fused echogenic thalami (t), and a relatively thin layer of parenchyma surrounding the single ventricle. (**c**) 3-D reconstruction of the cranium demonstrates the associated craniofacial deformities (microcephaly, hypotelorism, and cleft palate)

(1)   A single ventricle with separate occipital horns.
(2)   Fused thalami.
(3)   Partial development of the interhemispheric fissure and falx cerebri.
(4)   A small or absent third ventricle.
(5)   Normal cerebellum and brainstem.

## Semilobar holoprosencephaly

Semilobar is an intermediate form of holoprosencephaly with some division of the monoventricle into occipital and temporal horns. These children usually have significant intellectual retardation and only occasionally live beyond infancy[29]. Sonographic findings of semilobar holoprosencephaly[1,7,13,15] (Figure 8) include:

## Lobar holoprosencephaly

Lobar is the mildest form of holoprosencephaly, characterized by an absent septum pellucidum and frontal fusion. These patients have the longest

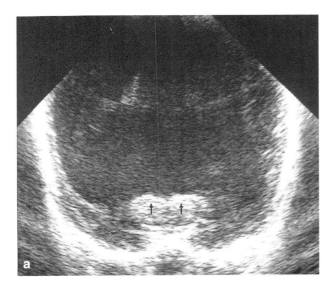

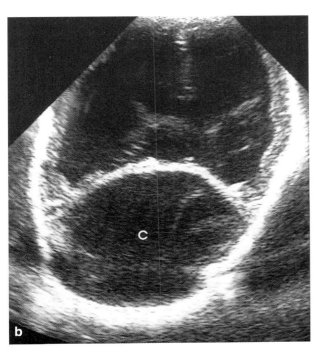

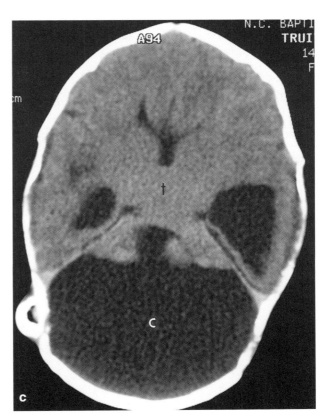

**Figure 7** Alobar holoprosencephaly associated with Dandy–Walker malformation. (**a**) Coronal view shows a massive monoventricle, fused echogenic thalami (t), and a thin rim of parenchyma surrounding the ventricle. (**b**) Another coronal image posteriorly demonstrates the monoventricle associated with a large posterior fossa cyst (c). (**c**) CT shows the fused thalami as well as agenesis of the cerebellar vermis and the fluid-filled posterior fossa

and agenesis of the corpus callosum with a midline cyst[30]. Also, lobar holoprosencephaly is similar sonographically to septo-optic dysplasia, and in fact, these entities may be part of the same spectrum of anomalies[12,30].

survival, but usually have severe mental retardation[29]. Sonographic findings of lobar holoprosencephaly include[13,15]:

(1) Absence of the septum pellucidum.
(2) Fusion of the frontal horns with squared, flat roofs and angular corners.
(3) Separate occipital horns.
(4) A shallow anterior interhemispheric fissure.
(5) Normal posterior interhemispheric fissure, thalami, and posterior horns.

Differential diagnostic considerations for holoprosencephaly should include hydranencephaly

## Absence of the septum pellucidum and septo-optic dysplasia

Absence of the septum pellucidum is easily identified by cranial sonography. However, the implications of that finding in terms of etiology and clinical consequences are much more complex. Absence of the septum pellucidum may occur as an isolated abnormality[31]. More commonly, however, it is a marker for other associated abnormalities of the brain, in which case there is usually some degree of neurologic impairment[31]. Examples of these include the Chiari II malformation,

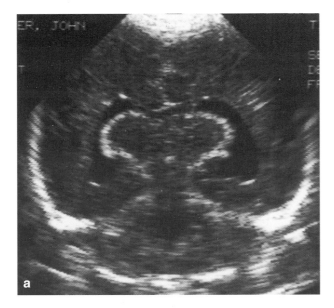

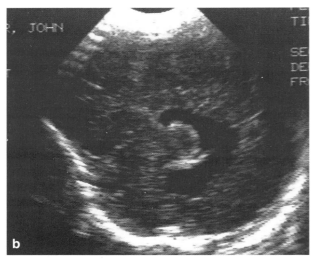

**Figure 8** Semilobar holoprosencephaly. (**a**) Coronal view shows a narrowly communicating monoventricle surrounding fused thalami and partial formation of the falx. (**b**) Right parasagittal view suggests some division of the monoventricle into separate temporal and occipital horns

holoprosencephaly, schizencephaly, agenesis of the corpus callosum, heterotopic gray matter, and encephaloceles[23,31].

When absence of the septum pellucidum is identified, another diagnostic consideration is the syndrome of septo-optic dysplasia (SOD), or DeMorsier syndrome, which is characterized structurally by absence of the septum pellucidum associated with hypoplasia of the optic nerves. Clinically, SOD causes deficiencies in ophthalmologic (decreased visual acuity, hypoplastic optic discs, nystagmus), neurologic (seizures, hypotonia),

and endocrinologic function (hypothyroidism, hypoglycemia, growth deficiency, diabetes insipidus)[1,12,13,15,32,33]. SOD may also be associated with cleft lip and palate, absence of the olfactory bulbs and tracts, schizencephaly, and partial absence of the corpus callosum[6,32,33].

Septo-optic dysplasia is a heterogeneous syndrome with great variability in its components. Barkovich *et al.*[34] recognize two subsets of septo-optic dysplasia with distinct associated features and embryologic origins: (1) SOD with schizencephaly, due to an early insult in the seventh or eighth week of development, and (2) SOD without schizencephaly, but with diffuse white matter hypoplasia, ventriculomegaly, and hypothalamic–pituitary dysfunction. This latter group may be a very mild form of lobar holoprosencephaly.

The diagnosis of septo-optic dysplasia requires the integration of clinical information with the anatomical information provided by imaging studies[34]. Therefore, given the appropriate clinical setting and a positive fundoscopic exam, sonography can suggest the diagnosis of septo-optic dysplasia[33].

## Sonographic findings

Sonographic findings of SOD[1,15,30–32] (Figure 9) include:

(1)  Absence of the septum pellucidum.
(2)  Box-like frontal horns, with inferior pointing at the thalamocaudate junction.
(3)  Dilatation of frontal and occipital horns of lateral ventricles. (The temporal horns are not dilated as in hydrocephalus.)
(4)  Enlarged anterior recess of the third ventricle.
(5)  Normal falx and interhemispheric fissure.

Septo-optic dysplasia should be distinguished from isolated absence of the septum pellucidum in which the frontal horns are usually less squared and no additional anomalies are identified clinically or sonographically[15]. Also, SOD is differentiated from lobar holoprosencephaly by the presence of atrophic optic nerves and normally separated frontal horns[1].

## Disorders of histogenesis, proliferation, and differentiation

### Vein of Galen malformation

The vein of Galen malformation is a large cerebral arteriovenous malformation which causes

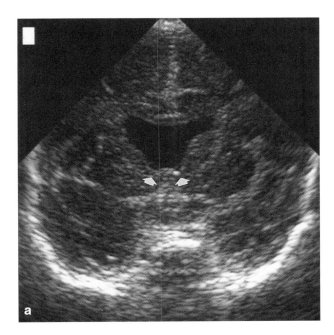

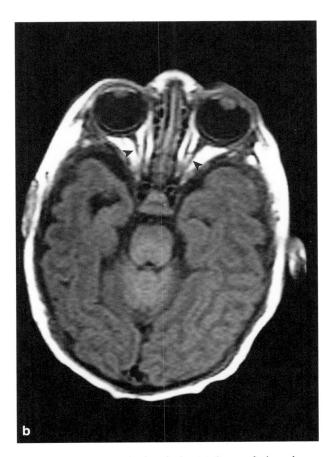

**Figure 9** Septo-optic dysplasia. (**a**) Coronal view shows absence of the septum pellucidum and box-like frontal horns with inferior pointing (arrows) at the thalamo-caudate junction. (**b**) MR axial image shows hypoplasia of the optic nerves (arrowheads)

aneurysmal dilatation of the vein of Galen[15]. The feeding arteries are anomalous branches of either the basilar or carotid circulation, with 90% of cases involving the posterior cerebral arteries[35]. The malformation is found in the region of the quadrigeminal plate cistern, and may cause secondary hydrocephalus due to a mass effect on the aqueduct of Sylvius[6,15]. Affected infants may present with high output congestive heart failure, cardiomegaly, cyanosis, prominent carotid pulsations, an enlarged head, a cranial bruit, seizures, or hemorrhage[1,6,7,15,36]. Treatment usually requires transcatheter embolization of the malformation[37]. Although prognosis is dependent on the timing and severity of presentation, long-term survival is rare[1,6,7].

Sonography is an especially useful modality for assessing the vein of Galen malformation, because it allows rapid diagnosis in the immediate postnatal period or in the critically ill infant, and it offers color Doppler analysis of flow[1–3,37–39]. It may be used both for preoperative mapping of the malformation and postoperative assessment of flow and effectiveness of embolization[40,41].

## Sonographic findings

Sonographic findings of the vein of Galen malformation[1,6,7,14,15,25,35,36,39,40] (Figure 10) include:

(1) Dilatation of the vein of Galen, which appears as a midline tubular mass in the region of the quadrigeminal plate cistern. It may be anechoic if filled with blood, or echogenic if filled with clot. Dilated feeding arteries and a dilated straight sinus posteriorly are also seen.
(2) Pulsation of the mass during real-time sonography.
(3) Increased flow and/or turbulence within the vein during color Doppler.
(4) Dilatation of the lateral ventricles due to hydrocephalus.
(5) Secondary parenchymal atrophy, periventricular leukomalacia, and calcification due to 'vascular steal' (decreased perfusion).

## Hydranencephaly

Hydranencephaly refers to the complete destruction of hemispheric parenchyma due to intrauterine bilateral occlusion or dysgenesis of the internal carotid arteries[25]. Although carotid

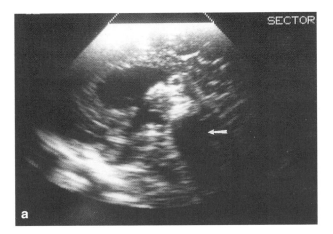

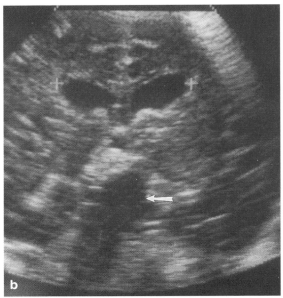

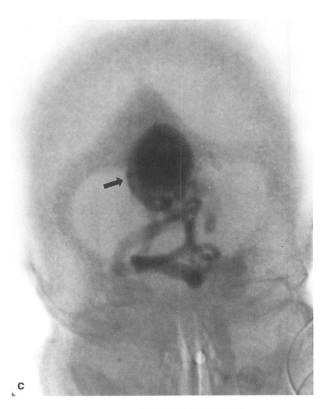

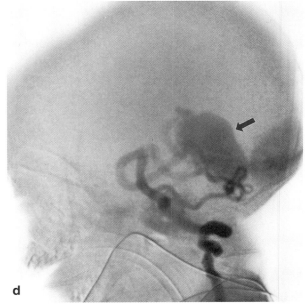

**Figure 10**   Vein of Galen malformation. (**a**) Sagittal and (**b**) coronal views demonstrate the dilated vein of Galen (arrow) posterior to the third ventricle. Note also the enlarged lateral ventricles indicating secondary hydrocephalus. (**c, d**) Cerebral arteriography via a left vertebral injection demonstrates the dilated vein of Galen (arrow) and its feeding arteries

occlusion is the generally accepted etiology, hydranencephaly has also been shown to be associated with toxoplasmosis, cytomegalovirus infection, and massive intracranial hemorrhage[2,3,42]. The cortical mantle and adjacent white matter is absent, replaced by a membranous sac containing CSF[15]. The areas of the brain supplied by the posterior circulation are intact, including the cerebellum, brainstem, parts of the occipital, frontal, and temporal lobes, thalami, hypothalamus, and basal ganglia[1,12,15,25]. True hydranencephaly is a nonviable condition[2,3].

## Sonographic findings

Sonographic findings of hydranencephaly[15] (Figure 11) include:

(1)   Absence of the cerebral hemispheres.
(2)   A large fluid-filled supratentorial cystic cavity.
(3)   Normal cerebellar hemispheres and thalami.
(4)   Intact falx cerebri.

Hydranencephaly should be differentiated from severe hydrocephalus, alobar holoprosencephaly, and severe bilateral subdural collections[43]. Using color Doppler, one can demonstrate the absence of the branches of the internal carotid arteries in hydranencephaly[43].

## Aqueductal stenosis

Aqueductal stenosis is the most common cause of congenital hydrocephalus[1]. Obstruction at the level of the aqueduct causes dilatation of the lateral and third ventricles which results in increased intracranial pressure. As a result, affected infants usually present with an enlarged head circumference.

Aqueductal stenosis is thought to be a disorder of proliferation, however it is difficult to classify as its pathogenesis remains uncertain[44]. The obstruction occurs in early intrauterine life, and may be congenital or acquired secondary to infection or hemorrhage[12]. Anatomically, the aqueduct may be either narrow and slit-like, or composed of multiple small channels which do not communicate with the ventricles or each other[44]. It is sometimes associated with other congenital abnormalities such as the Chiari II malformation and neurofibromatosis Type I[12].

## Sonographic findings

Sonographic findings of aqueductal stenosis[1] (Figure 12) include:

(1)    Dilatation of the lateral and third ventricles.
(2)    Normal size of the fourth ventricle.
(3)    Thinning of the cortical mantle.

## Hemimegalencephaly

Hemimegalencephaly, also known as unilateral megalencephaly, is a rare malformation of unknown etiology characterized by enlargement of part or all of one cerebral hemisphere with widened gyri, shallow sulci, and a thickened cortex[45,46]. Thickened white matter, heterotopic gray matter, and enlargement of the lateral ventricle on the megalencephalic side are also seen[45]. These infants present with a large head circumference, craniofacial asymmetry, early intractable seizures, mental retardation, and focal neurologic signs such as hemiplegia or

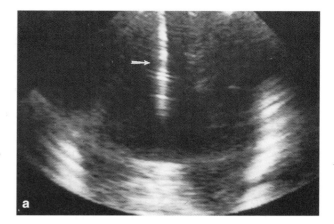

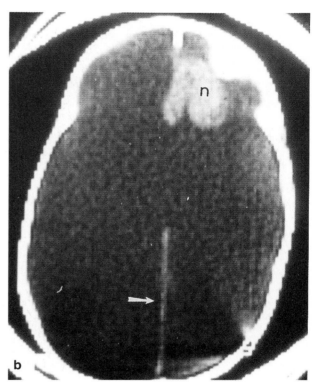

**Figure 11**  Hydranencephaly. (**a**) Coronal view demonstrates absence of cerebral parenchyma, which is replaced by an anechoic fluid-filled cavity. Note the intact falx (arrow). (**b**) CT demonstrates a fluid-filled supratentorial cavity with partial development of the falx (arrow) and a small amount of remaining neural tissue (n)

hemianopsia[45,46]. Some may also have hemihypertrophy of the body[47]. Hemimegalencephaly has a variable prognosis, ranging from death in the newborn period to survival into adulthood with some intellectual deficiency[45].

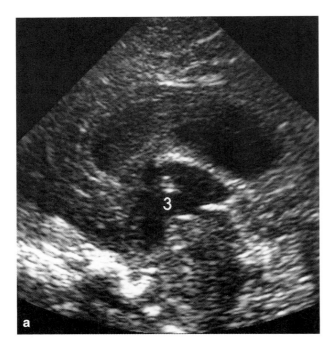

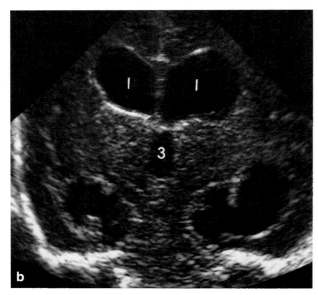

**Figure 12** Aqueductal stenosis. Midline sagittal view (**a**) and coronal view (**b**) in an infant with an enlarged head circumference shows massive dilatation of the lateral (1) and third (3) ventricles without enlargement of the fourth ventricle

## Sonographic findings

Sonographic findings of hemimegalencephaly[46–49] (Figures 13 and 14) include:

(1)  Enlargement of a cerebral hemisphere and its lateral ventricle.

(2)  Pachygyric ipsilateral cortex.
(3)  Widened and linear ipsilateral sylvian fissure.
(4)  Increased echogenicity of ipsilateral white matter.
(5)  Thickened gray matter with lack of gray–white matter interdigitation.
(6)  Shift of midline structures.

Note that despite the mass effect of hemimegalencephaly, the lateral ventricle remains enlarged and not compressed as might occur with neoplasm, hemorrhage, or edema[46]. This ventricular enlargement is anatomical and should not be confused with unilateral hydrocephalus[48].

## Disorders of migration

### Schizencephaly

Schizencephaly, or 'divided brain', is a rare malformation resulting in irregular, full-thickness clefts in the brain extending from the lateral ventricles to the cortical surface[15]. The clefts may be due to focal failure of the normal radial migration of neurons from the germinal matrix, or a temporary vascular occlusion in early intrauterine life causing a focal infarct of the germinal matrix[7,50]. The clefts are lined by cortical gray matter and are usually bilaterally symmetric[1,7,15]. They may be 'open-lipped' in which cerebrospinal fluid is contained in the cleft, or 'closed-lipped' in which there is no cerebrospinal fluid in the cleft[12,15].

Clinically, infants with schizencephaly often present with microcephaly, mental retardation, seizures, and developmental delay, including poor motor or speech development[15,51]. Unilateral closed-lip or small open-lip clefts have a good prognosis for intellectual development, whereas bilateral or large unilateral clefts have a poor prognosis[51].

## Sonographic findings

Sonographic findings of schizencephaly[1,7,13,15] (Figure 15) include:

(1)  Open fluid-filled clefts with echogenic edges communicating with the lateral ventricles. Closed clefts are difficult to identify with sonography.
(2)  Variable ventricular dilatation and dysmorphism.

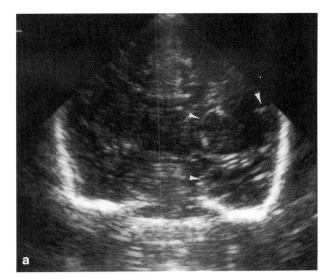

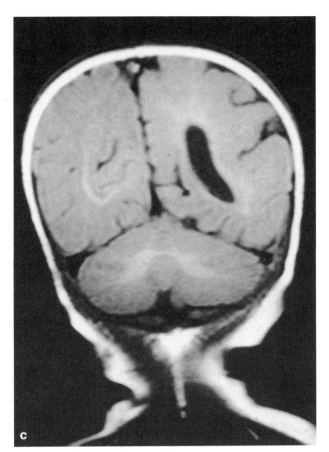

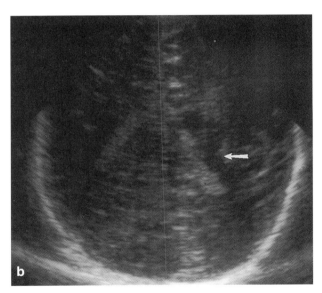

**Figure 13** Hemimegalencephaly. (**a**, **b**) Coronal views demonstrate asymmetric brain echogenicity, a larger, pachygyric left temporal lobe (arrowheads), and ipsilateral ventricular dilatation (arrow). (**c**, **d**) Coronal and axial MR images optimally demonstrate the pachygyric left cerebral cortex and ipsilateral ventricular dilatation

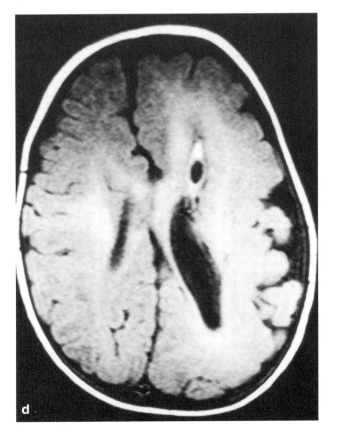

Other migrational disorders such as heterotopic gray matter, polymicrogyria, and agenesis of the corpus callosum are often associated and should be considered in cases of schizencephaly[1,7,13].

*Lissencephaly*

Lissencephaly, or 'smooth brain', is a rare disorder of sulcation and migration which results in an abnormal cortical mantle with failure to develop

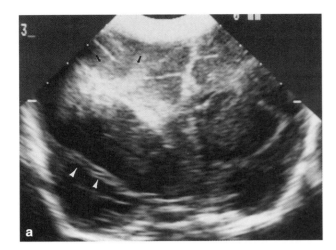

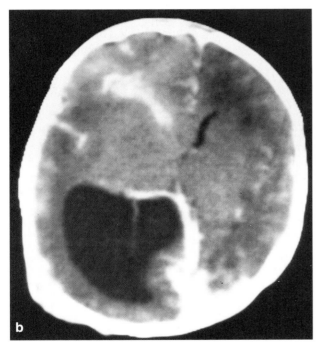

**Figure 14** Hemimegalencephaly. (**a**) Coronal view demonstrates a large right hemisphere with ipsilateral increased echogenicity of the white matter (arrows), shift of midline structures, and a linear sylvian fissure (arrowheads). Note that the right temporal lobe is enlarged compared to the left. (**b**) CT shows the degree of asymmetry between the right and left hemispheres in terms of size of the hemispheres, ventricular calibre, and gyral pattern

sulci or gyri[1,15]. Normally, in the third to sixth month of gestation, neuroblasts migrate radially from the subependymal germinal matrix to form the cerebral cortex. In lissencephaly, neuroblasts fail to migrate, resulting in a four-layered, instead of six-layered, cortex[15]. The malformation is usually symmetric and bilateral, and is characterized by microcephaly with enlarged ventricles, under-developed periventricular white matter, widened sylvian fissures, and minimal opercularization of the insula[1,13]. Lissencephaly may be associated with the Dandy–Walker complex, as well as other disorders of neuronal migration such as pachygyria, polymicrogyria, and heterotopic gray matter[52]. Infants with lissencephaly often have dysmorphic facial features, severe mental retardation, and seizures[53]. Death usually occurs within 18 to 24 months of birth[54].

## Sonographic findings

Sonographic findings of lissencephaly[7,15,53,54] (Figure 16) include:

(1)  Total or partial absence of gyri and sulci, i.e. a smooth brain.
(2)  Homogenous echotexture of the cerebral cortex.
(3)  Widened and linear sylvian fissures.
(4)  Widened subarachnoid space and large interhemispheric fissure.
(5)  Ventricular dilatation with colpocephaly.
(6)  Relative increase in periventricular echogenicity.

Although sonography is suggestive, MRI is the preferred modality for the diagnosis of lissencephaly. It is important to note that this malformation should not be confused with the normally smooth brain of the very premature infant, which develops a normal sulcal–gyral pattern over time[52].

### Agenesis of the corpus callosum

The corpus callosum normally forms in the third to fourth month of gestation as a bud from the lamina terminalis[1,7]. The callosal fibers cross the midline beginning anteriorly to form the genu and proceeding posteriorly to the splenium[23]. In complete agenesis of the corpus callosum (ACC), these fibers fail to cross the midline due to a vascular or inflammatory lesion of the commissural plate before the twelfth week of gestation[15]. Partial agenesis occurs when this developmental process is interrupted, resulting in absence of the corpus posteriorly[15,23]. Instead of crossing midline, the callosal fibers are directed longitudinally along the superomedial aspect of the lateral ventricles, creating so-called Probst's bundles[13,15].

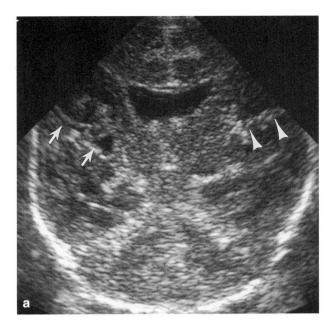

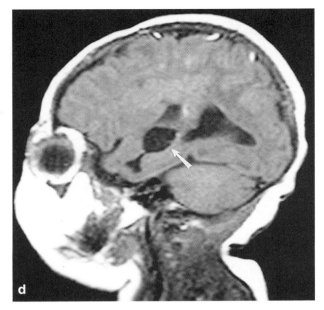

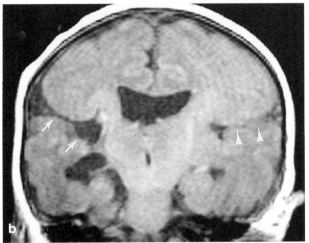

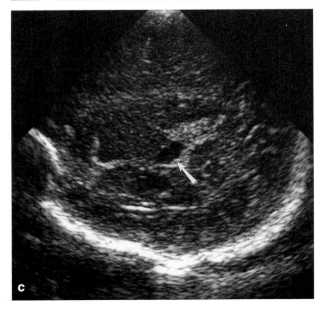

**Figure 15** Schizencephaly. Coronal US (**a**) and MR (**b**) images demonstrate bilateral schizencephalic clefts with the right larger than the left. On the ultrasound image, the open-lipped cleft on the right appears as an anechoic space extending peripherally (arrows). The closed-lipped cleft on the left is more subtle, as only the echogenic lining of the cleft is apparent (arrowheads). Note the associated absence of the septum pellucidum in this infant with septo-optic dysplasia. Sagittal US (**c**) and MR (**d**) images demonstrate the right-sided open-lipped cleft as an abnormal anechoic/hypointense space in the temporal lobe (arrow)

Agenesis of the corpus callosum may be isolated or may occur with associated anomalies. When isolated, ACC is usually asymptomatic, but may cause mental retardation and seizures[15,55]. Additional symptoms may be related to a wide variety of associated malformations, including interhemispheric arachnoid cysts and intracerebral lipomas, the Dandy–Walker complex, polymicrogyria, heterotopic gray matter, encephaloceles, Chiari II malformation, holoprosencephaly, septo-optic dysplasia, aqueductal stenosis, and porencephaly[1,7,8,42,55]. It is important to screen for these more significant anomalies when agenesis of the corpus callosum is identified[8].

## Sonographic findings

Sonographic findings of ACC[1,2,6,7,14,15,42,56] (Figure 17) include:

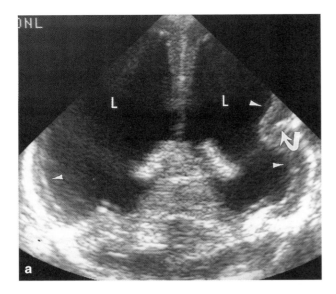

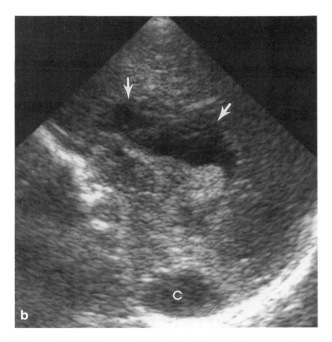

**Figure 16** Lissencephaly. (**a**) Coronal image shows massively enlarged lateral ventricles (L) with a thin rim of parenchyma and absence of gyri and sulci (arrowheads). The shallow sylvian fissure (curved arrow) gives a curved contour to the left lateral ventricle. (**b**) Sagittal view demonstrates the smooth, homogenous echotexture of the cerebral parenchyma. Note absence of the corpus callosum (arrows) and a posterior fossa cyst – Dandy–Walker variant (c)

(1) Partial or complete absence of the corpus callosum.

(2) Radial arrangement of the medial sulci around the roof of the third ventricle in a 'sunburst' or 'spoke wheel' pattern.

(3) Separation of frontal horns and bodies of the lateral ventricles.

(4) Dilatation and elevation of the third ventricle between the lateral ventricles.

(5) Sharply angled lateral peaks and concave medial borders of the frontal horns and bodies of the lateral ventricles. This shape yields a crescentic or horn-like appearance on coronal view.

(6) Colpocephaly.

Widening of the interhemispheric fissure and absence of the septum pellucidum are also commonly seen with ACC[2,13]. In addition, lipomas and interhemispheric cysts are often evident sonographically as brightly echogenic nodules and anechoic cysts, respectively[2,15].

## Conclusion

Cranial sonography has become the screening procedure of choice for the detection of CNS malformations in the neonatal nursery due to its practicality and versatility[2,3]. In contrast to CT or MRI, the challenge of sonography lies in developing the ability to recognize patterns of malformation without the exquisite tissue resolution available with more expensive and cumbersome modalities. With a working knowledge of the malformations presented and attention to the midline neuroanatomy, the major congenital brain malformations are readily identified with ultrasound. Furthermore, the detection of a congenital malformation should prompt a careful search for additional associated malformations.

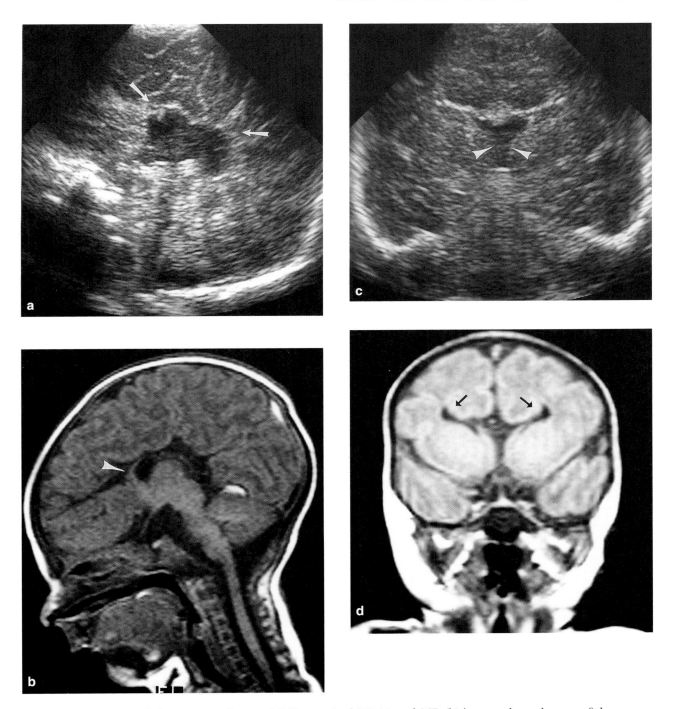

**Figure 17** Agenesis of the corpus callosum. Midline sagittal US (**a**) and MR (**b**) images show absence of the corpus callosum and radial arrangement of the medial sulci, giving the roof of the third ventricle an irregular contour (arrows). The MR shows near total agenesis, with a hypoplastic genu anteriorly (arrowhead). Coronal US (**c**) and MR (**d**) images reveal absence of the corpus callosum, enlargement and elevation of the third ventricle (arrowheads), dilatation of the foramen of Monro, and widely separated lateral ventricles with horn-like peaks and medial concavity (arrows) due to the protrusion of the Probst bundles

# References

1. Babcock DS. Cranial sonography: congenital anomalies. *Clinics in Diagnostic Ultrasound – Neonatal and Pediatric Ultrasonography* 1989;24:1–24

2. Grant EG, Tessler F, Perrella R. Infant cranial sonography. *Radiol Clin North Am* 1988;26:1089–110

3. Grant EG, White EM. Pediatric neurosonography. *J Child Neurol* 1986;1:319–37

4. Lipinski JK, Cremin BJ. Ultrasound and computed tomography of the infant brain: a clinical comparison. *Clin Radiol* 1986;37:365–9

5. Blickman JG, Jaramillo D, Cleveland RH. Neonatal cranial ultrasonography. *Curr Probl Diag Radiol* 1991;20:95–119

6. Levene MI. Non-cystic congenital abnormalities. *Clin Dev Med – Ultrasound Infant Brain* 1985;92:102–9

7. Babcock DS. Sonography of congenital malformations of the brain. *Neuroradiology* 1986;28:428–39

8. Gebarski SS, Gebarski KS, Bowerman RA, *et al.* Agenesis of the corpus callosum: sonographic features. *Radiology* 1984;151:443–8

9. Levene MI. Non-invasive assessment of neonatal cerebral function. *Dev Med Child Neurol* 1986;28:372–4

10. Siegel MJ, Patel J, Gado MH, *et al.* Cranial computed tomography and real-time sonography in full-term neonates and infants. *Radiology* 1983;149:111–16

11. van der Knaap MS, Valk J. Classification of congenital abnormalities of the CNS. *Am J Neuroradiol* 1988;9:315–26

12. Castillo M, Dominguez R. Imaging of common congenital anomalies of the brain and spine. *Clin Imaging* 1992;16:73–88

13. Rumack CM. Congenital brain malformations. In Rumack CM, Johnson ML, eds. *Perinatal and Infant Brain Imaging: Role of Ultrasound and Computed Tomography*. Chicago: Year Book Medical Publishers, 1984:91–115

14. Fischer AQ, Anderson JC, Shuman RM, *et al.* Malformations. In *Pediatric Neurosonography: Clinical, Tomographic, and Neuropathologic Correlates*. New York: John Wiley and Sons, 1985:199–230

15. Siegel MJ. Brain. In Siegel MJ, ed. *Pediatric Sonography*. New York: Raven Press, 1991:9–62

16. McLone DG, Naidich TP. Developmental morphology of the subarachnoid space, brain vasculature, and contiguous structures, and the cause of the Chiari II malformation. *Am J Neuroradiol* 1992;13:463–82

17. Diebler C, Dulac O. Cephaloceles: clinical and neuroradiological appearance. *Neuroradiology* 1983;25:199–216

18. McLone DG, Knepper PA. The cause of Chiari II malformation: a unified theory. *Pediatr Neurosci* 1989;15:1–12

19. Naidich TP, Altman NR, Braffman BH, *et al.* Cephaloceles and related malformations. *Am J Neuroradiol* 1992;13:655–90

20. Barkovich AJ, Kjos BO, Norman D, *et al.* Revised classification of posterior fossa cysts and cystlike malformations based on the results of multiplanar MR imaging. *Am J Neuroradiol* 1989;10:977–88

21. Osenbach RK, Menezes AH. Diagnosis and management of the Dandy–Walker malformation: 30 years of experience. *Pediatr Neurosurg* 1992;18:179–89

22. Altman NR, Naidich TP, Braffman BH. Posterior fossa malformations. *Am J Neuroradiol* 1992;13:691–724

23. Barkovich AJ. Congenital malformations of the brain and skull. In *Pediatric Neuroimaging*. New York: Raven Press, 1995:177–275

24. Mack LA, Rumack CM, Johnson ML. Ultrasound evaluation of cystic intracranial lesions in the neonate. *Radiology* 1980;137:451–5

25. Williams J. Intracranial cysts. *Clin Dev Med – Ultrasound Infant Brain* 1985;92:93–101

26. Chiou YM, Tsai CH. Axial sonographic features of Dandy–Walker variant with occipital cephalocele. *J Clin Ultrasound* 1992;20:139–41

27. Chilton SJ, Cremin BJ. Ultrasound diagnosis of CSF cystic lesions in the neonatal brain. *Br J Radiol* 1983;56:613–20

28. Fenichel GM. Disorders of cranial volume and shape. In *Clinical Pediatric Neurology: A Signs and Symptoms Approach*. Philadelphia: W.B. Saunders, 1993:361–78

29. Ashwal S. Congenital structural defects. In Swaiman KF, ed. *Pediatric Neurology: Principles and Practice*. St. Louis, MO: Mosby-Year Book, 1994:421–70

30. Fitz CR. Holoprosencephaly and related entities. *Neuroradiology* 1983;25:225–38

31. Kuhn MJ, Swenson LC, Youssef HT. Absence of the septum pellucidum and related disorders. *Comput Med Imag Graphics* 1993;17:137–47

32. Kuban KCK, Teele RL, Wallman J. Septo-optic-dysplasia-schizencephaly: radiographic and clinical features. *Pediatr Radiol* 1989;19:145–50

33. Nowell M. Ultrasound evaluation of septo-optic dysplasia in the newborn: report of a case. *Neuroradiology* 1986;28:491–2

34. Barkovich AJ, Fram EK, Norman D. Septo-optic dysplasia: MR imaging. *Radiology* 1989;171:189–92

35. Stockberger S, Smith R, Don S. Color Doppler sonography as a primary diagnostic tool in the diagnosis of vein of Galen aneurysm in a critically ill neonate. *Neuroradiology* 1993;35:616–18

36. Jones RWA, Allan LD, Tynan MJ, *et al.* Ultrasound diagnosis of cerebral arteriovenous malformation in the newborn. *Lancet* 1982;1:102–3

37. Schimmel MS, Bruckheimer E, Hammerman C. Neonatal radiology casebook: neonatal symptoms of vein of Galen aneurysmal malformation. *J Perinatol* 1994;14:325–7

38. Sivakoff M, Soraya N. Diagnosis of vein of Galen arteriovenous malformation by two-dimensional ultrasound and pulsed Doppler method. *Pediatrics* 1982;69:84–6

39. Snider AR, Soifer SJ, Silverman NH. Detection of intracranial arteriovenous fistula by two-dimensional ultrasonography. *Circulation* 1981;63:1179–85

40. Cohen HL, Haller JO. Advances in perinatal neurosonography. *Am J Radiol* 1994;163:801–10

41. Westra SJ, Curran JG, Duckwiler GR, *et al.* Pediatric intracranial vascular malformations: evaluation of treatment results with color Doppler US. *Radiology* 1993;186:775–83

42. Kendall BE. Dysgenesis of the corpus callosum. *Neuroradiology* 1983;25:239–56

43. Doi H, Tatsuno M, Mizushima H, *et al.* The use of two-dimensional Doppler sonography (color Doppler) in the diagnosis of hydranencephaly. *Child Nerv Syst* 1990;6:456–8

44. Roessmann U. Congenital malformations. In Duckett S, ed. *Pediatric Neuropathology*. Philadelphia: Williams and Wilkins, 1995:123–48

45. Kalifa GL, Chiron C, Sellier N, *et al.* Hemimegalencephaly: MR imaging in five children. *Radiology* 1987;165:29–33

46. Lam AH, Villanueva AC, de Silva M. Hemimegalencephaly: cranial sonographic findings. *J Ultrasound Med* 1992;11:241–4

47. Sandri F, Pilu G, Dallacasa P, *et al.* Sonography of unilateral megalencephaly in the fetus and newborn infant. *Am J Perinatol* 1991;8:18–20

48. Babyn P, Chuang S, Daneman A, *et al.* Sonographic recognition of unilateral megalencephaly. *J Ultrasound Med* 1992;11:563–6

49. Fariello G, Malena S, Lucigrai G, *et al.* Hemimegalencephaly: early sonographic pattern. *Pediatr Radiol* 1993;23:151–2

50. Suchet IB. Schizencephaly: antenatal and postnatal assessment with color-flow Doppler imaging. *Can Assoc Radiol J* 1994;45:193–200

51. Barkovich AJ, Kjos BO. Schizencephaly: correlation of clinical findings with MR characteristics. *Am J Neuroradiol* 1992;13:85–94

52. Trounce JQ, Fagan DG, Young ID, *et al.* Disorders of neuronal migration: sonographic features. *Dev Med Child Neurol* 1986;28:467–71

53. Motte J, Gomes H, Morville P, *et al.* Sonographic diagnosis of lissencephaly. *Pediatr Radiol* 1987;17:362–4

54. Cioffi V, Bossi MC, Ballarati E, *et al.* Lissencephaly in two brothers detected by US: A 'pseudo-liver' pattern. *Pediatr Radiol* 1991;21:512–14

55. Byrd SE, Radkowski MA, Flannery A, *et al.* The clinical and radiological evaluation of absence of the corpus callosum. *Eur J Radiol* 1990;10:65–73

56. Babcock DS. The normal, absent, and abnormal corpus callosum: sonographic findings. *Radiology* 1984;151:449–53

# Sonography in periventricular leukomalacia and intraventricular hemorrhage

*Roger S. Yang and Harris L. Cohen*

Modern technology has allowed the survival of greater and greater numbers of premature infants. Many of these infants will suffer spastic motor deficits later in life with an incidence as high as 15%[1-6]. Prominent intellectual deficits and developmental disabilities can be seen in as many as half of these infants. Intraventricular hemorrhage (IVH) and periventricular leukomalacia (PVL) are thought to be the major neuropathologic causes of these brain injuries and their sequelae in premature infants.

Evaluation of the premature brain for abnormality begins with and often ends with ultrasonography. Other diagnostic tools such as computed tomography (CT), magnetic resonance imaging (MRI), and rarely cerebral angiography are also useful in evaluating the infant brain but are far less often utilized. The popularity of ultrasound hinges in large part on its portability, lack of ionizing radiation, and relatively low cost. Ultrasound is the predominant screening tool for IVH and PVL in the premature infant with or without demonstrated signs of neuropathology[7]. Recognized limitations in sonography include some blind areas along the convexities (particularly close to the vertex) and the lack of a global view of the brain which could be more readily provided by CT and MRI.

Recognition of patients at risk for IVH, PVL, and their sequelae as well as the timing of their examination are vital to their care and treatment. Most lesions can be identified within the first weeks of life[2,8]. Questionable areas can be followed on a periodic basis as clinically indicated. Due to the prevalence of this disease in the premature and low birth weight infant, some neonatal intensive care units will screen all patients less than 1500 g and less than 32 weeks gestation at birth. Such infants are under significant clinical stresses and are at particular physiologic risk for the development of IVH, PVL, and their sequelae.

Recent studies seem to indicate that MRI is the most sensitive study in the detection of these intracranial lesions. However, due to the relative difficulty in obtaining magnetic resonance examinations of premature infants on ventilators and to the cost of MRI scanning, screening by MRI is impractical. In addition, an experienced sonographer or sonologist can piece imaged sectors into a complete view of the brain. Ultrasound can create images in coronal and longitudinal planes using the various fontanelles and calvarial sutures as sonographic windows. Transcranial views using lower frequency transducers can produce axial images even through the calvarium itself. Doppler and color Doppler allow rapid assessment of lesions for vascularity. Small cystic abnormalities that may be beyond the resolution of CT may be seen only by ultrasound. Interestingly, ultrasound is more sensitive in detecting PVL than is CT[3,9].

## Intraventricular hemorrhage

IVH is the most common intracranial lesion of the premature infant. The incidence seems to be directly related to the degree of prematurity. The incidence of this disease entity in infants less than 1500 g and less than 32 weeks gestation has been reported to range between 25 and 40%[8,10-12]. The incidence seems to be decreasing, with current reports noting numbers at the lower end of this range. However, due to the larger numbers of lower birth weight infants surviving the premature period, IVH continues to be a serious and often-diagnosed clinical problem. Most of these lesions (over 80%) will be detectable within the first three days and certainly by the end of the first week of life[13-18]. Therefore, unless the clinical picture requires emergent sonographic examination, it has been suggested that an initial scan should be performed between the fourth and seventh days of life[18]. Follow-up sonograms for the sequelae of any lesions identified on the first scan are typically performed one or two weeks later[18]. Clinical findings and symptomatology such as spastic motor and intellectual deficits increase in direct proportion to the severity of the hemorrhage.

## Pathogenesis

IVH originates predominantly from germinal matrix area hemorrhages. The germinal matrix is a band of tissue present during fetal life and found in the subependymal area at the floor of the body and temporal horn of the lateral ventricles. The largest mass of germinal matrix is found at the junction of the head of the caudate nucleus and the thalamus. This area is known as the caudo-thalamic groove (Figure 1) and is readily seen on sagittal ultrasound images. The germinal matrix does not extend into the occipital horn.

The germinal matrix is made up of spongio-blasts and neuroblasts that will eventually give rise to mature elements of neural tissue in the cortex and basal ganglia. The germinal matrix is not normally seen in term infants. It can still be noted in the premature infant. By six months gestation most of the germinal matrix has involuted. At about 24 weeks (the borderland of neonatal viability), the germinal matrix consists of only a small area of cells situated in the caudo-thalamic groove. The tissue is supported by a large number of vessels whose vascular endothelium is one cell layer thick. These vessels are therefore friable and prone to injury. If bleeding occurs, the structures surrounding the germinal matrix are at risk for cell injury and destruction and the patient is at risk for significant neurologic injury.

Germinal matrix area hemorrhages can be locally limited to the subependymal area but they may also extend into the ventricular system[12]. When blood enters the cerebrospinal fluid (CSF) of the ventricular system it may clot and obstruct the ventricles locally. It may create hematoma beyond the foramina of Luschka or Magendie. The blood may exit the ventricles and create an arachnoiditis secondary to the subarachnoid heme (usually at the pacchionian granulations) leading to the typical extraventricular post-hemorrhagic hydrocephalus.

The pathogenesis of subependymal/germinal matrix and intraventricular bleeds seems multi-factorial. Volpe has elegantly subdivided these into extravascular, intravascular, and vascular causes[12].

The extravascular factors Volpe describes in the pathogenesis of IVH are deficiencies in the supportive tissues around the vasculature. The germinal matrix area is a gelatinous, friable structure with many large and fragile capillary and arteriolar vessels within it. The supporting mesenchymal structure seems insufficient to fully stabilize and protect the vessels and thus there is a propensity to hemorrhage. Active fibrinolytic

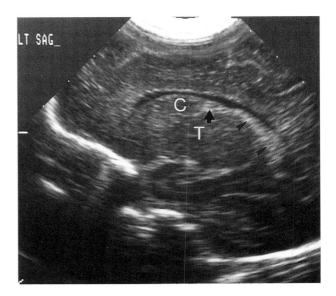

**Figure 1** Normal parasagittal view. Left parasagittal plane. The caudate head (C) and the thalamus (T) are seen. An arrow points to the caudothalamic groove. Cerebrospinal fluid is seen as anechoic fluid within a non-dilated ventricle. Arrowheads point to choroid plexus within the lateral ventricle

activity is characteristically found in developing organ systems and the germinal matrix is no exception. The actions of the fibrinolytic enzymes contribute to further weakening in the supporting structure of the germinal matrix.

Intravascular factors contributing to the pathogenesis of germinal matrix bleeds center on fluctuations in cerebral blood flow. There appears to be at least a subset of premature infants who have difficulty stabilizing intracerebral arterial flow in the setting of varying systemic arterial pressures. These patients have what is defined as a pressure passive intracerebral arterial system that, unlike that of adults, is not pressure sensitive and whose vessels do not adjust to changes in systemic blood pressure. The pressure passive system predisposes the infant to germinal matrix bleeds. Widely varying systemic pressures found in premature infants on mechanical ventilation as well as during other forms of physiologic distress may be enough to provoke a germinal matrix bleed. However, the major factor that causes changing intracerebral arterial pressures is brain ischemia. Hypercapnia from RDS and other forms of respiratory distress will result in preferential blood flow to the brain. Without compensatory vascular changes to control the pressure intracranially, distention of the friable germinal matrix vessels may cause them to break and a bleed to occur. Increases in the cerebral venous pressure as noted in the stresses of labor and delivery, perinatal asphyxia, and pneumothorax can increase venous pressure leading to intracerebral vessel distention and subsequent bleeding. Alternatively, decreases in cerebral blood flow may cause ischemic damage to the delicate germinal matrix vessels.

Vascular factors that predispose the germinal matrix to hemorrhage essentially relate to the immaturity of the vessels in the germinal matrix. The cells that make up the vessels are in the process of remodeling and thus are intrinsically weak. These vessels are therefore prone to ischemic damage. Upon reperfusion after an ischemic injury, these already weak vessels may readily rupture.

The controversy over pathogenesis of what was classically described as grade IV IVH will be explored later in this chapter.

## Sonographic findings of IVH

### Grade I

Subependymal hemorrhage, germinal matrix hemorrhage, and grade I intraventricular hemorrhage are all terms used to refer to bleeding confined to the germinal matrix area without any intraventricular extension (Figure 2). Neurosonographically, these bleeds may be imaged as echogenic areas at the caudothalamic groove. They may be seen on coronal images just lateral to the frontal horns at the caudothalamic groove. They may involve the entire caudate head. Grade I hemorrhages (as with all grades of IVH) may be unilateral or bilateral. This type of hemorrhage is usually asymmetric[19].

Subependymal hemorrhages may resolve entirely over a matter of days. Some grade I bleeds will leave only a small echogenicity as a remnant[20]. Many lesions will liquefy over time and can be imaged as a cystic lesion or lesions in the area of hemorrhage (Figure 3). This can remain present for months before resolution. The purely cystic lesions appear no different on ultrasound from subependymal cysts reported in association with non-hemorrhagic ischemia or infection or those of unknown origin. Post-hemorrhagic ventriculomegaly from grade I IVH develops in approximately 5% of these patients[21].

### Grade II

Subependymal hemorrhage that extends into but does not distend the lateral ventricles is labeled

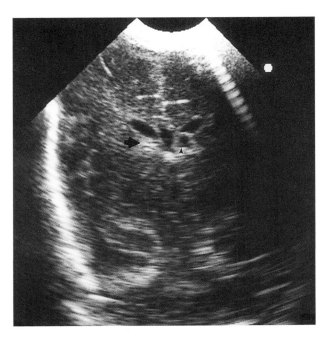

**Figure 2** Grade I intraventricular hemorrhage and subependymal cyst. Coronal view. An echogenic subependymal hemorrhage is seen on the right side (arrow). An echoless subependymal cyst is seen on the left side (arrowhead). This represents residua from a prior hemorrhage

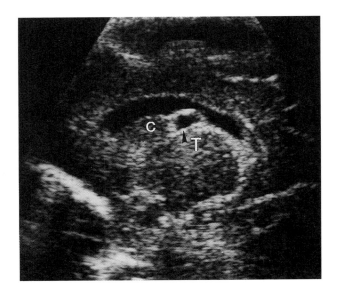

**Figure 3** Germinal matrix cyst. Left parasagittal view. At the caudothalamic groove between the head of the caudate (C) and the thalamus (T), there is a cystic area that represents a germinal matrix cyst (arrowhead). In this patient with previously imaged grade I subependymal hemorrhage, this is the residua of the hemorrhage. Cysts may also be seen on the basis of germinolysis from intrauterine infection or other intrauterine insult

grade II intraventricular hemorrhage. This is visualized sonographically as hyperechogenicity within a non-dilated ventricle (Figure 4). It may be difficult to differentiate this grade of IVH from an isolated germinal matrix bleed (Grade I IVH) that abuts the ventricle. However, this differentiation does not have great clinical significance as the prognoses for both grade I and grade II IVH are good to excellent.

Acute hemorrhage is as brightly echogenic as the normal choroid. This may pose a diagnostic dilemma when hemorrhage is found within the lateral ventricles as in grades II–IV IVH. However, if there is bright echogenicity within the ventricle that is anterior to the foramen of Munro, then this definitively represents hemorrhage since choroid plexus is invariably located posterior to the foramen of Munro. Another useful point in

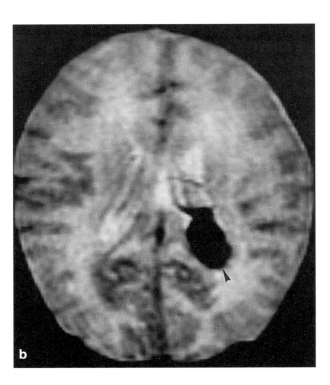

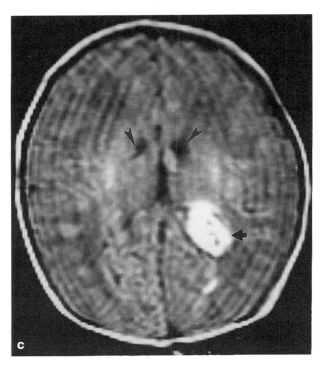

**Figure 4** Grade II intraventricular hemorrhage (IVH) (**a**) Coronal view. Normally echogenic choroid is seen in a non-dilated right ventricle (C). The echogenic area in the left lateral ventricle is asymmetric and represents choroid plexus and equally echogenic hemorrhage adjacent to it (H). No significant ventricular dilatation is seen. (**b**) MRI axial view of T2 weighted image. This MRI scan confirms the grade II IVH noted in (**a**). Low signal area (arrowhead) in the region of the atrium of the lateral ventricle is consistent with hemorrhage. Bright signal within the non-dilated lateral ventricles is consistent with CSF. The ventricles are not enlarged. (**c**) MRI axial view of T1 weighted MRI. Intraventricular hemorrhage is seen as a high signal area within the atrium of the left lateral ventricle (arrow) and corresponds to the low signal area noted previously on the axial T2 weighted MRI image. The frontal horns of the lateral ventricles are noted bilaterally (arrowheads) and are of normal size, suggesting grade II IVH

differentiating blood from normal choroid plexus is the normal anterior tapering of the choroid compared with the more bulbous shape of the typical intraventricular hemorrhage. Comparison with the contralateral side cases of grade II IVH may demonstrate asymmetry. Unfortunately, in a small, slit-like ventricular system, small amounts of intraventricular blood may be difficult to identify. More often the hemorrhage will dilate the ventricular system. There is then a semantics problem in distinguishing between grade II and grade III IVH.

Complete resolution with little or no ventriculomegaly is the usual sequela of grade II bleeds. As mentioned, progression of the bleed with developing ventriculomegaly can also result. Blood can circulate through the CSF to eventually result in arachnoiditis and its complications. Ventricular dilatation after resolution of the grade II bleed has been said to be seen in about 25% of such patients[21].

## Grade III

Intraventricular extension of germinal matrix hemorrhage with ventricular dilatation is labeled grade III IVH. The ultrasound diagnosis is easier in this grade due to the readily recognizable blood or clot in dilated ventricles. In the acute setting, the echogenic mass-like lesion within the enlarged ventricle is usually seen somewhere in the body of the lateral ventricles (Figures 5 and 6). As previously stated, echogenicity anterior to the foramen of Munro can distinguish blood from normal choroid. Blood–CSF levels can sometimes be seen in dependent portions. It can extend to fill almost the entire ventricular space which will give the ventricles an appearance of being filled with dense echogenicity without any identifiable anechoic CSF. The blood can fill the third and fourth ventricles. Grade III IVH is often bilateral and can be symmetric.

The intraventricular blood typically will resorb and decrease in echogenicity as the clot naturally ages and fibrin levels within the clot decrease. Fragmentation can result as the clot begins to retract. Retracted clot often has an echogenic margin with a more echopenic central mass (Figure 7). As the clot retracts, CSF will be seen around the periphery of the clot. Some element of ventriculomegaly will usually persist after resolution of the clot (which may take an average of about six weeks). Those patients with post-hemorrhagic ventriculomegaly represent about

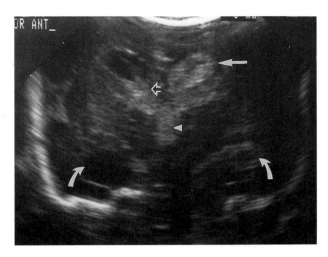

**Figure 5** Grade III intraventricular hemorrhage. Coronal view. Clot is noted within a somewhat dilated left frontal horn (arrow). Echogenicity noted in the third ventricle is consistent with acute hemorrhage (arrowhead). The temporal horns are somewhat dilated (curved arrows) with the right containing no clot and with the left containing echogenicity which probably represents clot. The small echogenic area seen within the right frontal horn (open arrow) may represent choroid plexus or, less likely, clot of a different age

55% of grade III bleeds. Fibrotic bands or septae can sometimes be identified within the echoless intraventricular CSF as residua of this hemorrhage[21].

## Grade IV

Before description of the sonographic findings of grade IV IVH (intraventricular hemorrhage with hemorrhage in a dilated ventricle and also seen in the brain parenchyma), the pathogenesis of periventricular hemorrhagic infarctions and necrosis will be discussed as there appears to be a relationship between intraventricular hemorrhage and periventricular hemorrhagic infarctions. For many years it was theorized that hemorrhage could extend directly into the brain parenchyma from the subependymal area. Over the last several years, Volpe has suggested that this hemorrhage may lead to an associated venous infarction and brain destruction simulating a direct extension of the hemorrhage[5,12,22–27]. Volpe's theory is based on the temporal difference of two days seen between IVH and the associated intraparenchymal hemorrhage[28]. Many of the parenchymal hemorrhages previously labeled grade IV hemorrhage

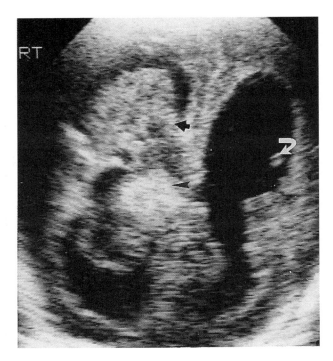

**Figure 6** Grade III intraventricular hemorrhage. Coronal view. The lateral ventricles are significantly dilated. There is clot seen in the right lateral ventricle (arrow) with some relatively echopenic areas within it that suggests that it is not an acute clot. The brighter echogenicity seen (arrowhead) probably represents more acute hemorrhage or hemorrhage that has not yet undergone liquefaction. The left lateral ventricle contains some debris within it (curved arrow) related to hemorrhage

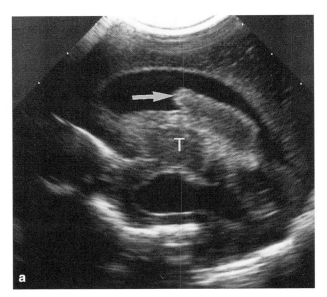

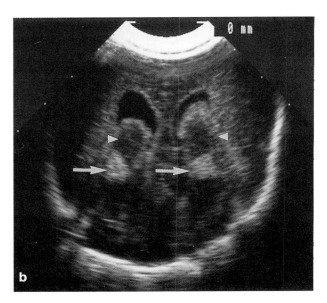

**Figure 7** Subacute grade III intraventricular hemorrhage. Subacute state. (**a**) Right parasagittal view. An echogenic structure is seen in a moderately dilated left lateral ventricle. It is relatively echopenic except for its somewhat bright periphery (arrow). The above is the clot retraction that is typically seen in an aging clot with retraction. There is a more echopenic central area with continued peripheral echogenicity. The clot's image will evolve until eventual dissolution. T, thalamus. (**b**) Coronal view. The lateral ventricles are moderately dilated. The bright echogenicity seen in both lateral ventricles (arrows) represents choroid plexus. The more echopenic structures with peripheral echogenicity seen anteriorly are subacute intraventricular clots (arrowheads)

may be a result of venous infarction and subsequent hemorrhage. Some authors feel that the original and classic theory of parenchymal extension from intraventricular hemorrhage is not the predominant pathogenetic mechanism in grade IV hemorrhage. There is evidence that there is at least an association between intraventricular hemorrhage (of any grade) and periventricular hemorrhage[27].

The pathogenetic mechanism of periventricular infarction and subsequent hemorrhage is thought to involve the following: (1) intraventricular hemorrhage occurs; (2) intraventricular blood causes increased ventricular pressure which subsequently decreases periventricular flow; (3) there is a local release of physiologically irritative factors upon the vasculature; and (4) there may be physical blockage by the hemorrhage of local terminal venous flow from thrombosis or destruction of the draining veins as they cross into the area of intraventricular bleed[27]. Therefore, parenchymal blood theoretically may be explained on the basis of hemorrhagic infarction caused by intraventricular hemorrhage rather than parenchymal extension of an intraventricular hemorrhage.

Whatever the pathogenetic mechanism, the grade IV IVH is the most clinically serious of the forms of IVH. Hemorrhage seen in the brain parenchyma defines this lesion. Ipsilateral ventriculomegaly and intraventricular blood is a common associated finding. The intraparenchymal component is imaged sonographically as a lesion of increased echogenicity usually in the frontal or parietal periventricular areas (Figures 8 and 9). The size of the intraparenchymal lesion varies from small punctate foci to a massive parenchymal hemorrhage extending to the periphery of the cortex. Asymmetry of involvement is not uncommon even when the grade IV IVH is bilateral. Differentiation between this lesion and similar appearing periventricular ischemic lesions (from PVL) may be difficult. In differentiating grade III from grade IV IVH, one should attempt to discern purely intraventricular blood from parenchymal blood directly adjacent to the ventricle.

The grade IV IVH may regress over a period of several weeks with clot retraction and eventual clot dissolution. During this period of time, the intraparenchymal hemorrhage may initially liquefy and appear as a hypoechoic area with a well defined rim. Internal echogenicity may represent residual areas of clot as it retracts and fragments. Eventually, these areas of intraparenchymal hemorrhage will become cystic. They are usually few in number and large in size. They may be a single large cystic area of porencephaly that communicates with the ventricle. This will not disappear over time. Eventually the area involved will atrophy. Ventricular dilatation following grade IV hemorrhage will develop in 80% of cases[21].

## Prognosis

Major spastic motor deficits are the major sequelae to subependymal and intraventricular hemorrhage. These deficits are often in the form of spastic hemiplegia. As these hemorrhages are often unilateral, the motor loss will often be unilateral. If the symptoms are bilateral, they are often asymmetric in severity. Unlike the bilateral spastic diplegia of periventricular leukomalacia, the spastic hemiplegia of IVH will involve both the upper and lower extremities as there is

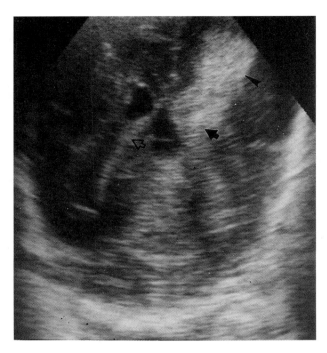

**Figure 8** Grade IV intraventricular hemorrhage. Coronal view. Bright echogenicity consistent with acute hemorrhage is seen within the left lateral ventricle (arrow). This area seems to extend into the parenchyma of the left frontal brain (arrowhead). Arrowheads point to normal right lateral ventricle with contained choroid plexus (open arrow). Current theory states that this is not hemorrhagic extension but rather coexistent periventricular infarction as the cause of the appearance of this image

concomitant damage to the descending corticospinal tracts from both upper and lower motor cortices. Intellectual deficits are included in the spectrum of neurologic sequelae of IVH. For patients with grade I IVH, significant neurologic or intellectual deficits have been reported in 15%. The percentage rises to 30% for grade II IVH, 40% for grade III IVH and is as high as 90% for grade IV IVH[20,21,29].

Mortality rises in direct proportion to the severity of the intraventricular hemorrhage. Patients with grade I bleeds have a reported 15% mortality rate. Patients with grade II suffer 20% mortality. Mortality rates for grade III and grade IV IVH are 40% and 60% respectively[21].

## Periventricular leukomalacia

PVL is an ischemic abnormality seen in prematurity that is thought to be a cause of spastic

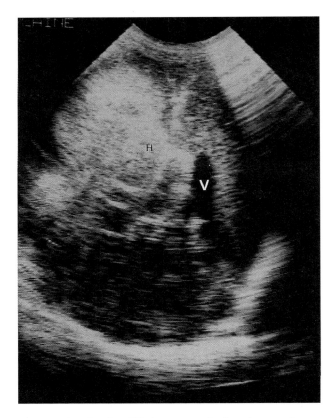

**Figure 9** Grade IV intraventricular hemorrhage. Coronal view. Another example of grade IV hemorrhage shows a highly echogenic area in the right brain that obscures the right lateral ventricle (H). Mildly to moderately dilated left lateral ventricle (V) is seen

diplegia and prominent neurologic deficits. The incidence in low birth weight infants has been measured at anywhere from 12% to 40%[9,30–32]. It is especially common in premature infants who have suffered severe cerebral hypoxia or cardiopulmonary distress.

The parenchyma is injured and is imaged as abnormal in characteristic arterial watershed distribution areas in the deep white matter dorsal and lateral to the external angles of the lateral ventricles. This will begin to lead to encephalomalacia with cavity and cyst formation in the area of pathology. Months later, the affected area may fill in with gliosis. Ultrasonographic imaging will show no abnormality after gliosis occurs despite the presence of histologically abnormal brain.

PVL and IVH are commonly associated. Not only is hemorrhage seen in upwards of 59% of cases, but approximately 36% of IVH patients will exhibit findings of PVL[33–35]. The ischemic lesions may demonstrate intrinsic hemorrhage in about

25% of autopsy cases although most of these lesions seen at autopsy are not necessarily seen on imaging studies[36]. Generally, the smaller the lesion, the less likely it is to be hemorrhagic.

## Pathogenesis

Theories as to the pathogenesis of PVL are somewhat similar to those of subependymal hemorrhage. Again, the pressure passive cerebral circulation seen in the premature neonate will render the patient susceptible to decreases in arterial flow. Decreased systemic arterial pressure will translate into decreased cerebral pressures. The areas where leukomalacia are commonly seen are those that are particularly susceptible to injury from decreased blood flow. Specifically, these are the watershed regions between the major arterial supply distributions within the brain. The immature and actively differentiating glial cells of the premature brain are inherently at greater risk for injury from ischemia. This is especially true in the periventricular area where cells also exhibit anaerobic glycolysis that leads to the build up of harmful lactic acid and to the depletion of intracellular energy supplies[27].

## Sonographic appearance of PVL

PVL presents in its acute phase as areas of increased echogenicity lateral to the frontal horns and trigones of the lateral ventricles (Figure 10). The hyperechogenicity is reported as bilateral in one-half of the cases. The lesion varies in contour from being small and curvilinear to large, broad, and coarse areas of hyperechogenicity. One must take care to differentiate the normal periventricular echogenic halo or 'blush' that is seen in infants from PVL, as both present sonographically as increased periventricular echogenicity. However, the normal periventricular 'blush' is said to be usually less well-defined than the PVL lesion[37] (Figure 11).

After approximately two weeks the true periventricular leukomalacia lesions will undergo cystic degeneration. The cysts are typically anechoic with a variably thick rim of echogenicity (Figure 12). They are usually multiple and can have the appearance of a cyst with multiple septations (Figure 13). When the PVL lesion is small, it is less likely that one will sonographically image its cystic degeneration. The larger lesions in PVL will almost invariably demonstrate cystic degeneration.

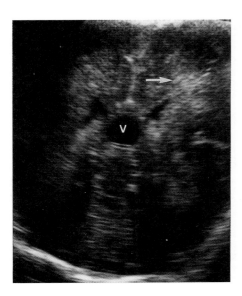

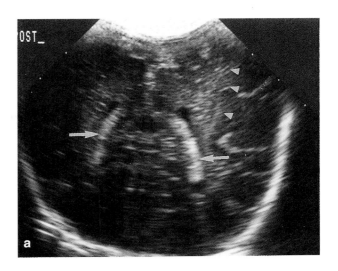

**Figure 10** Periventricular leukomalacia (PVL). Acute echogenic state. Coronal view. There is asymmetric echogenicity of the white matter superior and lateral to the frontal horn. This can sometimes be technical. In this case, follow-up images showed cyst development at this site proving the bright echogenicity on the left (arrow) to be acute PVL. The normal cavum vergae extension of the cavum septum pellucidum is noted as 'V'

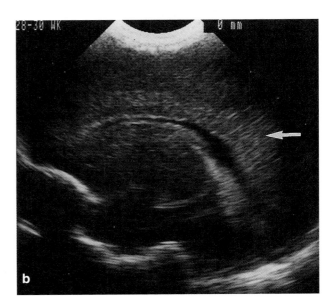

The development of cysts confirms the diagnosis of PVL.

The areas of cystic degeneration may calcify. The multicystic appearance may persist to varying degrees but will usually resolve sonographically over a span of a few months. Diffuse cerebral atrophy and ventriculomegaly can be the long term imaging findings of PVL.

*Prognosis*

Premature infants with PVL will demonstrate spastic diplegia, seizures, and sensory deficits as their major neurologic sequelae. Less severe developmental and intellectual deficits will also be seen.

As opposed to grade IV hemorrhage, where degrees of unilateral hemiplegia are more common, PVL is often associated with bilateral neurologic involvement. In PVL, the decrease in intracerebral blood pressure will affect watershed zones bilaterally whereas IVH will tend to be more unilateral and asymmetric. The periventricular regions that are injured in PVL correspond to the

**Figure 11** Normal periventricular echogenicity. (**a**) Coronal view. The lateral ventricles are normal in size. Arrows point to normal choroid plexus within the lateral ventricles. Arrowheads point to bright periventricular echogenicity that appears relatively symmetric. This is most often normal. The increased echogenicity is thought to be a result of anisotropic effect on white matter fibers. As discussed, this may simulate acute periventricular leukomalacia. (**b**) Normal periventricular echogenicity. Right parasagittal view. Anisotropic effect is probably the reason for normal increased echogenicity seen just posterior to the atrium of the left lateral ventricle (arrow) in the posterior watershed area

more medial corticospinal tracts and therefore result in prominent lower extremity neurologic deficits known as spastic diplegia[27]. The degree of neurologic symptomatology from this lesion is

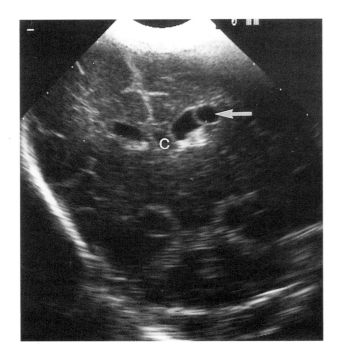

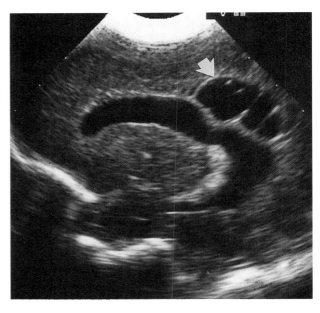

**Figure 13**   Periventricular leukomalacia (PVL). Cystic stage. Right parasagittal view. A moderately dilated lateral ventricle is noted. Several cysts (arrow) are noted in the brain parenchyma superior to the posterior body of the ventricle. This is consistent with posterior watershed cystic PVL. Arrowheads point to the choroid plexus

**Figure 12**   Periventricular leukomalacia (PVL). Cystic stage. Coronal view. Mildly dilated frontal horns of the lateral ventricles are noted. A large cyst (arrow) has developed in the anterior watershed region which in this case appears to have some mass impression on the frontal horn. Cyst development in an area of previously noted increased echogenicity in either the anterior or posterior watershed areas is diagnostic for PVL. Cavum septum pellucidum is marked with a 'C'

directly related to the severity and size of the lesion[20,27]. PVL is associated with low mortality rates but significant morbidity.

Ultrasound has great uses in intracranial diagnosis of the premature infant at risk for IVH,

PVL and their sequelae. Increasing experience with this imaging tool and adjunctive imaging methods should provide us with greater abilities to aid our perinatal colleagues in the management of the premature infant.

# References

1. Calame A, Fawer CL, Claeys V, *et al*. Neurodevelopmental outcome and school performance of very low birth weight infants at 8 years of age. *Eur J Pediatr* 1986;145:461–6
2. Fawer CL, Diebold P, Calame A. Periventricular leukomalacia and neurodevelopmental outcome in preterm infants. *Archiv Dis Child* 1987;62:30–6
3. Blennow G, Pleven H, Lindroth M, Johanssen G. Long-term follow-up of ventilator treated low birth-weight infants. *Acta Paediatr Scand* 1986;75:827–31
4. Stewart A, Hope PL, Hamilton P, *et al*. Prediction in very preterm infants of satisfactory neurodevelopmental progress at 12 months. *Dev Med Child Neurol* 1988;30:53–63
5. Volpe JJ. Brain injury in the premature infant – current concepts of pathogenesis and prevention. *Biol Neonate* 1992;62:231–42
6. Radack DM, Baumgart S, Gross GW. Subependymal (grade 1) intracranial hemorrhage in neonates on extracorporeal membrane oxygenation. Frequency

and patterns of evolution. *Clin Pediatr* 1994;33: 583–7

7. Carson SC, Hertzberg BS, Bowie JD, *et al*. Value of sonography in the diagnosis of intracranial hemorrhage and periventricular leukomalacia: a postmortem study of 35 cases. *Am J Radiol* 1990;155: 595–601

8. Paneth N, Pinto-Martin J, Gardiner J, *et al*. Incidence and timing of germinal matrix/intraventricular hemorrhage in low birth weight infants. *Am J Epidemiol* 1993;137:1167–76

9. Keeney SE, Adcock EW, McArdle CB. Prospective observations of 100 high-risk neonates by high-field (1.5 Tesla) magnetic resonance imaging of the central nervous system. *Pediatrics* 1991;87:431–8

10. Levene MI, Wigglesworth JS, Dubowitz V. Hemorrhagic periventricular leukomalacia in the neonate: a real-time ultrasound study. *Pediatrics* 1983;71:794–7

11. Papile LA, Burstein J, Burstein R, *et al*. Incidence and evolution of subependymal and intraventricular hemorrhage: A study of infants with birth weights less than 1500 gm. *J Pediatr* 1978;92:529–34

12. Volpe JJ. Intraventricular hemorrhage in the premature infant – current concepts. Part I. *Ann Neurol* 1989;25:3–11

13. Rumack CM, Manco-Johnson ML, Manco-Johnson MJ, *et al*. Timing and course of neonatal intracranial hemorrhage using real-time ultrasound. *Radiology* 1985;154:101–5

14. Dolfin T, Skidmore MB, Fong DK, *et al*. Incidence, severity and timing of subependymal and intraventricular hemorrhages in preterm infants born in a perinatal unit as detected by serial real-time ultrasound. *Pediatrics* 1983;71:541–6

15. Levene MI, Fawer CL, Lamong RF. Risk factors in the development of intraventricular hemorrhage in the pre-term neonate. *Arch Dis Child* 1982;57: 410–17

16. Partridge JC, Babcock DS, Steichem JJ, *et al*. Optimal timing for diagnostic cranial ultrasound in low birthweight infants: detection of intracranial hemorrhage and ventricular dilatation. *J Pediatr* 1983;102:281–7

17. Perlman JM, Volpe JJ. Intraventricular hemorrhage in extremely small premature infants. *Am J Dis Child* 1986;140:1122–4

18. Timor-Tritsch IE, Monteagudo A, Cohen HL. *Ultrasonography of the Prenatal and Neonatal Brain*. Stamford: Appleton & Lange, 1996:269–74

19. Perlman JM, Rollins N, Burns D, *et al*. Relationship between periventricular intraparenchymal echodensities and germinal matrix-intraventricular hemorrhage in the very low birth weight neonate. *Pediatrics* 1993;91:474–80

20. Siegel MJ. Intracranial hemorrhage: Brain. In Siegel MJ, ed. *Pediatric Sonography*. New York: Raven Press, 1991:18–25

21. Shankaran S, Slovis TL, Bedard MP, *et al*. Sonographic classification of intracranial hemorrhage. A prognostic indicator of mortality, morbidity, and short-term neurologic outcome. *J Pediatr* 1982;100: 469–75

22. Volpe JJ. Brain injury in the premature infant: diagnosis, prognosis, and prevention. *Clin Perinatol* 1989;16:387–411

23. Babcock D, Han B. *Cranial Ultrasonography of Infants*. Baltimore: Williams & Wilkins, 1981:140–235

24. Grant E, Borts F, Schellinger D, *et al*. Real-time ultrasonography of neonatal intraventricular hemorrhage and comparison with computed tomography. *Radiology* 1981;139:687–91

25. Grant E. Neurosonography: germinal matrix-related hemorrhage. In Grant E, ed. *Neurosonography of the Pre-term Neonate*. New York: Springer-Verlag, 1986: 33–68

26. Takashima S, Mito T, Ando Y. Pathogenesis of periventricular white matter hemorrhages in preterm infants. *Brain Dev* 1986;8:25–30

27. Volpe JJ. Current concepts of brain injury in the premature infant. *Am J Radiol* 1989;153:243–51

28. Cohen HL, Haller JO. Advances in perinatal neurosonography. *Am J Radiol* 1994;163:801–10

29. Volpe JJ. Intracranial hemorrhage: periventricular-intraventricular hemorrhage of the premature infant. In Volpe JJ, ed. *Neurology of the Newborn*, 2nd edn. Philadelphia: W.B. Saunders, 1987:311–61

30. Pape KE, Armstrong DL, Fitzhardinge PM. Central nervous system pathology associated with mask ventilation in the very low birthweight infant: a new etiology for intracerebellar hemorrhage. *Pediatrics* 1976;58:473–81

31. Larroche JC. Hypoxic brain damage in fetus and newborn. Morphologic characters. Pathogenesis. Prevention. *J Perinatal Med* 1982;10(S):29–31

32. Skullerud K, Westre B. Frequency and prognostic significance of germinal matrix hemorrhage, periventricular leukomalacia, and pontosubicular necrosis in preterm neonates. *Acta Neuropathol* 1986;70:257–61

33. Schellinger D, Grant EG, Richardson JD. Cystic periventricular leukomalacia: sonographic and CT findings. *Am J Neuroradiol* 1984;5:439–45

34. Shuman RM, Selednik LJ. Periventricular leukomalacia. A one year autopsy study. *Neurology* 1980; 37:231–5

35. McMenamin JB, Shackelford GD, Volpe JJ. Outcome of neonatal intraventricular hemorrhage with periventricular echodense lesions. *Ann Neurol* 1984;15:285–90

36. Armstrong D, Norman MG. Periventricular leukomalacia in neonates: complications and sequelae. *Arch Dis Child* 1974;49:367–75

37. DiPietro MA, Brody AB, Teele RL. Peritrigonal echogenic 'blush' on cranial sonography: pathologic correlates. *Am J Radiol* 1986;146:1067–72

# Ultrasound of the neonatal gastrointestinal tract  4

*Susan C. D. Comerci and Terry L. Levin*

Sonographic evaluation of the infant gastrointestinal tract (including Doppler ultrasound) has gained increasing acceptance over the past decade. It is well tolerated by infants, as well as their parents. Its bedside mobility for infants on life-supportive devices has added to its popularity[1,2].

Obtaining a technically good ultrasound examination of an infant often poses a challenge; anatomy is in constant motion and increased bowel gas can obscure underlying structures[3]. Ensuring that the infant is warm and comfortable is essential. A pacifier may be all that is necessary to soothe the infant. Alternatively, the exam can be performed while the infant is being fed, if clinically appropriate, or immediately following a feeding. Scanning with a slow and steady motion of the transducer may be better tolerated than inconstant contact of the transducer with the infant's abdomen[4]. Anticipating the infant's respiratory motion will aid in obtaining static images. If bowel gas obscures anatomy, administering fluids into the stomach can create an ultrasonic window and allow improved visualization of underlying structures. A window can also be improved by pushing bowel gas away with gentle pressure or by repositioning the infant.

## Esophagus

Using a subxiphoid approach to the abdomen, the distal esophagus is visualized anterior to the aorta at the level of the diaphragm, although it is often overlooked. Sonographically, it is a tubular structure with a thin sonolucent outer muscular wall, surrounding collapsed echogenic mucosa and submucosa. Additional portions of the esophagus can be visualized through alternative approaches such as suprasternal, parasternal, subcostal, or subxiphoid approaches[5].

### Gastroesophageal reflux

Gastroesophageal reflux (GER), a common disorder in infants, often presents with vomiting. While most cases resolve spontaneously, rarely, GER may cause failure to thrive, irritability, unusual posturing, esophagitis, chronic anemia, esophageal stricture, recurrent pneumonia, wheezing, and apnea[6–8].

Several imaging modalities may be used to detect GER. The contrast upper gastrointestinal study detects reflux occurring at the time of the exam, provides anatomic detail of the esophageal mucosa, and identifies associated abnormalities such as hiatal hernia, stricture, esophagitis, and aspiration. Gastroesophageal scintigraphy (which images over time) is more sensitive in detecting GER[6]. Extended esophageal pH monitoring is the most sensitive technique to detect reflux[7].

Although ultrasound may be performed for the investigation of reflux, most often reflux is noted while performing the exam for another indication. When GER is sonographically imaged, opening of the lower esophageal sphincter and retrograde flow of gastric contents may be seen. The echogenicity of the refluxed material depends on the relative amounts of fluid and gas. Competency of the lower esophageal sphincter, length of the intra-abdominal portion of the esophagus, gastroesophageal angle, and the presence or absence of a sliding esophageal hiatus may be identified. In addition, the examiner may observe associated clinical symptoms while reflux is occurring[8].

## Stomach

The body and antrum of the stomach are visualized through the epigastric area with the infant in a supine position. The antropyloric region is best visualized with the patient in a right lateral decubitus position. The stomach should be filled with fluid to accurately assess wall thickness as lack of gastric distension may cause apparent wall thickening. A small amount of fluid in the antrum enables improved visualization of the pylorus.

The gastric antrum is anterior to the pancreas and has a target appearance. The mucosa and submucosa make up the inner echogenic layer; the outer muscular layer is hypoechoic. Fluid contents provide an anechoic center. The normal thickness of the stomach wall is 3 mm or less[9].

Multiple conditions may cause increased gastric wall thickness. These include Henoch-Schonlein purpura, ectopic pancreas, gastric ulceration, lymphoid hyperplasia, gastritis, Crohn's disease, and chronic granulomatous disease[10]. Thickening may be smooth or irregular, symmetric or asymmetric.

## Focal foveolar hyperplasia

Focal foveolar hyperplasia (FFH) is a non-neoplastic mucosal polyp that occurs in the stomach in adults, and rarely in children. The fovea, which normally compose approximately half the thickness of the mucosal layer, are the pits in the mucosa into which the gastric glands empty. In FFH, these pits elongate, widen and become tortuous, resulting in a papillary appearance which forms a broad-based polyp. This may cause partial gastric outlet obstruction, presenting with vomiting. Superficial erosions may result in bleeding[11,12].

FFH presenting as gastric outlet obstruction has been reported in ductal dependent neonates on prostaglandin $E_1$[13]. Prostaglandin $E_1$ has been shown to induce proliferation of the gastric antral mucosa causing elongation and dilatation of the gastric pits[14]. The condition is related to duration of therapy and cumulative dose of prostaglandins. Newborns who receive prostaglandin $E_1$ at the recommended dose of 0.05 $\mu$g kg$^{-1}$ min$^{-1}$ for more than 120 hours are at greatest risk. The hyperplasia appears to be reversible, regressing after cessation of the drug[13]. On ultrasound, marked increased thickening of the echogenic mucosal layer of the gastric antrum is seen (Figures 1a, b and 2a, b).

## Microgastria

During the fifth fetal week, the stomach forms as a dilatation of the caudal portion of the foregut. It rotates 90 degrees clockwise and moves toward the left. The posterior portion of the stomach grows more rapidly than the anterior portion, forming greater and lesser curvatures[15].

Microgastria is a rare congenital anomaly that results when the stomach fails to undergo normal growth and rotation, resulting in a small tubular stomach without a distinct fundus[15,16]. It is associated with other anomalies (related by

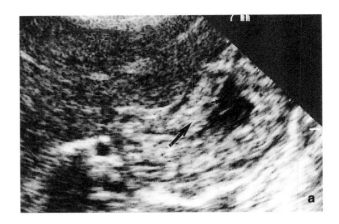

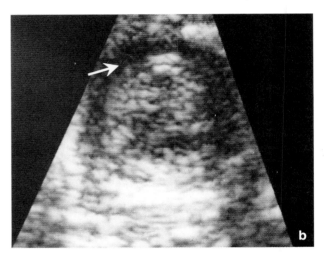

**Figure 1** (**a**) Ultrasound of the stomach in a 1-month-old, ex-24 week premature infant on prostaglandin therapy. There is marked thickening of the echogenic mucosa (large arrow). The central echo-poor area represents fluid in the gastric lumen (small arrow). (**b**) Transverse ultrasound through the gastric antrum in the same patient. Marked thickening of the central echogenic mucosa is present. The echo-poor rim (arrow) represents the other layers of the gastric wall

location and timing in embryologic growth), which include malformations of the heart, lungs, gastrointestinal tract, and asplenia. The esophagus is usually markedly dilated and elongated, presumably as an adaptation to compensate for the small storage capacity of the underdeveloped stomach[15-17]. Ultrasound reveals a small, usually midline, tubular stomach, and may reveal asplenia, a transverse liver, and other associated abnormalities (Figure 3a,b).

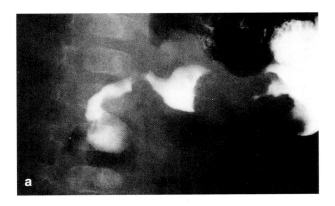

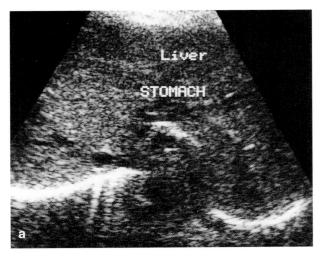

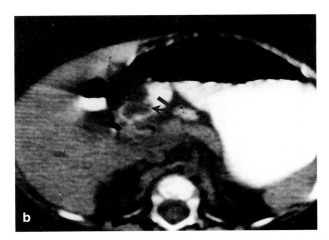

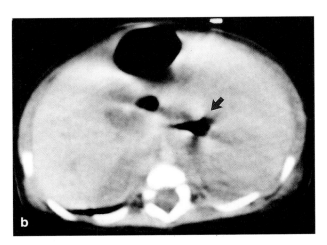

**Figure 2** (**a**) Spot film from an upper gastrointestinal tract series in a 3-month-old male on high-dose prostaglandin therapy. The gastric antrum and pyloric region are markedly narrowed by antral mucosal hyperplasia simulating pyloric stenosis. (**b**) CT of the upper abdomen in the same patient demonstrates a focal area of mucosal hyperplasia in the gastric antrum (arrow) presenting as an antral mass

**Figure 3** (**a**) Transverse ultrasound through the upper abdomen in a newborn with multiple congenital abnormalities. The stomach is tiny. Note the transverse appearance of the liver in this infant with microgastria, situs ambiguous and asplenia. (**b**) CT in the same patient. The air filled stomach is tiny (arrow). The liver is transverse. (The large anterior air filled structure was found to be a Meckel's diverticulum at surgery)

## Antral web

Antral web is a congenital remnant, which may represent a failure of complete recanalization of the gastric lumen or it may be the result of an ischemic event *in utero*. Its presence causes a relative gastric outlet obstruction, presenting with vomiting or failure to thrive. Although less frequent, it may mimic hypertrophic pyloric stenosis. Sonographically, it may be visualized as a persistent echogenic structure crossing the prepyloric region. The stomach may be dilated proximally. The pylorus is normal. The antrum should be distended with fluid to exclude redundant gastric mucosa and should be imaged over time to exclude a peristaltic wave[18].

## Gastric duplication

Gastric duplications are rare. They are usually located along the greater curvature and most do not communicate with the gastric lumen. They may cause distension or pain, and may ulcerate. Sonographically they appear as simple cysts adjacent to the gastric lumen (Figure 4). They may have solid echogenic portions representing hemorrhage or inspissated material. The wall of the cyst has a characteristic anechoic peripheral rim, corresponding to the smooth muscle layer,

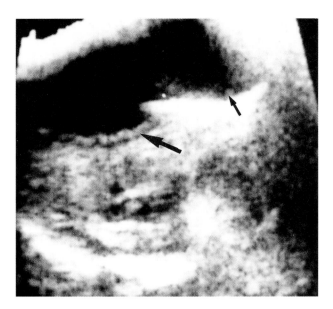

**Figure 4** Upper abdominal ultrasound in a newborn with vomiting. There is an anechoic fluid filled duplication cyst (large arrow) adjacent to the fluid filled stomach (small arrow). Note the echogenic mucosal layer and echo-poor muscle layer ('double wall sign')

and an inner echogenic mucosal layer. This forms the 'double wall sign' (see discussion on duplication cysts)[19,20].

## Lactobezoar

A lactobezoar may form when an infant is fed powdered formula which has not been adequately diluted. A non-specific hyperechoic mass may be seen by ultrasound. Administering water may help demonstrate that the mass is intraluminal[21].

## Gastric emptying

Ultrasound has been used to measure the volume of fluid present in the stomach. Although nuclear scintigraphy is the method of choice in evaluating gastric emptying, if repeated at timed intervals, ultrasound can be used as a gross estimate of gastric emptying. Unlike nuclear scintigraphy, in which fluids and solids are individually labeled, ultrasound can not differentiate between these components[22].

## Duodenum

### Hypertrophic pyloric stenosis

Hypertrophy of the circular muscle of the pylorus is an acquired condition which narrows the pyloric canal[23]. Signs and symptoms include dehydration, vigorous gastric peristalsis, and non-bilious vomiting. Infants usually present with symptoms between 2 and 6 weeks of age. The incidence of hypertrophic pyloric stenosis (HPS) is approximately 3 in 1000, with a male-to-female ratio of 5 : 1[1].

The hypertrophied muscle can often be diagnosed when palpated as an olive-shaped mass in the epigastrium (about 80% of cases) and is treated by surgical pyloromyotomy[24,25]. When the clinical findings are unclear, sonography has largely replaced the upper gastrointestinal series (UGI) in the diagnosis of HPS.

Many of the classical UGI findings in HPS, such as the beak sign, the string sign, and the shoulder sign of the hypertrophied muscle indenting the antrum, are also demonstrable by ultrasound[26,27]. In addition, ultrasound provides direct visualization of the pyloric muscle.

The infant is placed in the right posterior oblique position which aids in the visualization of the pylorus. If there is not enough residual gastric fluid present, 60 to 120 ml of water may be administered either orally or through a nasogastric tube. The stomach should not be overfilled, as this displaces the pylorus posteriorly, making visualization more difficult[28].

The hypertrophied muscle has a typical appearance on ultrasound. On short-axis view the pylorus resembles a 'bull's-eye' or 'target' with the thickened hypoechoic peripheral muscle surrounding the central echogenic mucosa. On long-axis view, the muscle is thickened, elongated and extends into the antrum; this appearance has been called the 'cervix' sign by Ball (a term originally used by Schuster in the endoscopic diagnosis of adult HPS)[29] (Figure 5a,b). If fluid passes through the pyloric canal, it is often seen as a 'double-track' in the crevices of the compressed mucosa, similar to the appearance on UGI[30]. Exaggerated gastric peristalsis, delayed gastric emptying and GER (originally described in the UGI) are also helpful secondary signs which may be seen on ultrasound.

The pyloric muscle frequently has a non-uniform echo pattern, with the near and far fields appearing more echogenic. This artifact, known as the anisotropic effect, is caused by the incidence of

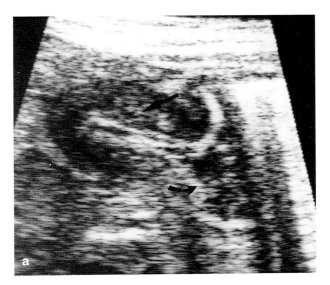

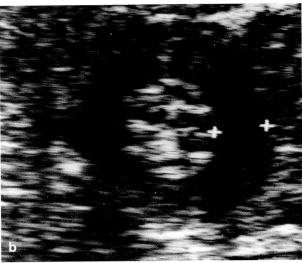

**Figure 5** (a) Longitudinal ultrasound of pylorus in a 4-week-old male with vomiting. The pyloric muscle (large arrow) is markedly thickened (curved arrow, antrum). (b) Transverse ultrasound of the pylorus in the same infant with hypertrophic pyloric stenosis. The pylorus has a target appearance. The markers denote the thickened echo-poor pyloric muscle

the ultrasound beam relative to the orientation of the circular muscle fibers[28,31].

Sonographic measurement of pyloric muscle thickness enables the diagnosis of HPS. Measurements must be carefully obtained along long and short axes. If the image is oblique, measurements will be overestimated. A muscle thickness of 4 mm or greater on the long-axis view is a reliable indicator of HPS (Blumhagen)[32,33]. Others use a muscle thickness of 3 mm or greater as the diagnostic measurement for HPS (O'Keefe)[9], a channel length of 17 mm or greater (Stunden),

and pyloric muscle length of 20 mm or greater (Wilson & Vanhoutte). The least reliable measurement is the transverse serosal-to-serosal diameter, which is considered abnormal if it is 15 mm or greater (Strauss). Some have advocated the use of pyloric volume to diagnose HPS (Westra)[34].

The differential diagnosis includes pylorospasm, gastrointestinal reflux, and duodenal obstruction due to stenosis or malrotation with bands or volvulus[27].

### Duodenal atresia/stenosis/web

Obstruction of the duodenum causes proximal duodenal dilatation. Causes of duodenal obstructions include atresia, stenosis, web, or annular pancreas. Ultrasound may demonstrate large fluid filled tubular structures representing the dilated stomach and proximal duodenum. Lack of duodenal distension may occur after vomiting[35].

## Small bowel

### Malrotation/volvulus

Malrotation with midgut volvulus, a surgical emergency, should be considered in any infant with bile-stained vomiting. Malrotation occurs when normal *in utero* rotation of the bowel does not proceed. The midgut is fixed on a short mesentery, and is prone to twisting around the axis of the superior mesenteric artery (SMA). When volvulus occurs, the vascular supply to the bowel is compromised and total infarction of the midgut may occur. The UGI examination remains the gold standard in the diagnosis of malrotation. However, one should be aware of the ultrasonographic signs of malrotation, especially when malrotation has not been considered clinically.

The superior mesenteric vein (SMV) normally lies to the right of the SMA. Malrotation may be suggested on ultrasound if the superior mesenteric vein is to the left or anterior to the artery[36,37] (Figures 6a,b and 7). However, this is neither a specific nor a sensitive sign. In one series of infants with malrotation studied by ultrasound, the position of the SMA and SMV were inverted in 67% and normal in 33%. In one patient in whom volvulus had already occurred, the vessels were normally positioned[36]. In another study (Dufour *et al.*), malrotation was present in all cases where the SMV was to the left of the SMA. However, malrotation also occurred when the SMV was

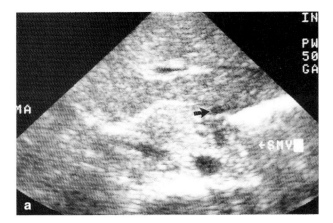

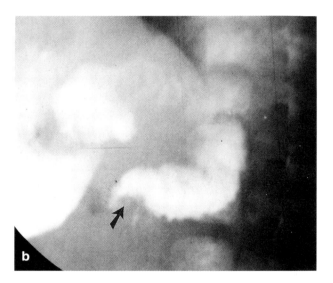

**Figure 6** (a) Transverse ultrasound of the abdomen in a 4-day-old with bilious vomiting. The superior mesenteric vein is to the left of the superior mesenteric artery (arrow). (b) Spot film from an upper gastrointestinal tract series in a newborn with bilious vomiting. There is an abrupt cut off of the duodenum. Note the beaked appearance of the duodenum (arrow) in this patient with midgut volvulus

anterior to the SMA or normally related to the SMA in a small number of cases. While an abnormal position of the SMV to SMA may raise the suspicion of malrotation, a normal relationship of the SMV to SMA does not exclude malrotation[37].

A more specific sign for malrotation with midgut volvulus is the sonographic 'whirlpool' sign, reported by Pracros. The superior mesenteric vein and mesentery are visualized as a 'whirlpool' around the SMA[35]. Smet *et al.* described hyperkinetic pulsations in the SMA, located in the center of the volvulated bowel. The SMV could not be identified, probably due to compression[38].

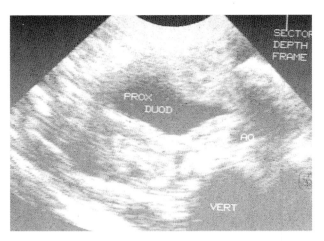

**Figure 7** Transverse ultrasound of the dilated proximal duodenum in a patient with midgut volvulus. The duodenum comes to a 'beak' at the point of twist

Other suggestive but less reliable signs of malrotation include the distended, fluid-filled proximal duodenum or an abnormal course of the duodenum[39,40]. It should be emphasized that a UGI should be performed in all patients in whom malrotation is suspected.

### Duplications

Enteric duplications may occur anywhere in the gastrointestinal tract. As described in the previous section on gastric duplications, they may appear sonographically as simple cysts or may appear solid and echogenic due to hemorrhage or inspissated material. Duplications may be suggested by ultrasound by demonstrating the 'double wall sign' which represents the echogenic mucosal layer of the cyst and the anechoic peripheral smooth muscle layer (Figures 8a,b and 9a,b). The two layers are often difficult to see circumferentially on any single image, but using multiple images, can usually be seen in at least 50% of the cyst wall. This double wall appearance has not been described with any other type of cyst, and is felt to be pathognomonic for enteric duplication[41].

### Jejunal/ileal atresia

Small bowel atresias result from an ischemic event that occurs *in utero*. Sonographically, large fluid filled structures representing bowel loops may be imaged. Extraluminal echogenic foci may be visualized if accompanying meconium peritonitis is present (Figures 10 and 11a,b).

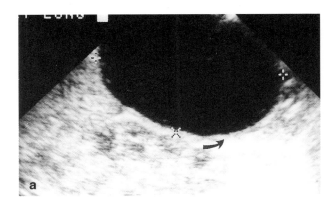

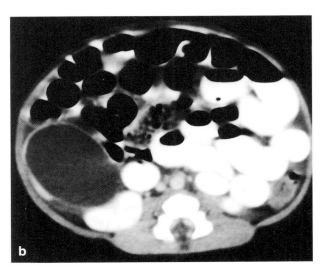

**Figure 8** (**a**) Ultrasound of the right lower quadrant in a newborn with right flank mass. A cystic structure with an echogenic lining (arrow) is present. (**b**) CT in the same patient. The cystic mass is anterior and extrinsic to the right kidney. At surgery, this was an ileal duplication

## Meconium ileus

In 10% of patients with cystic fibrosis, meconium ileus presents as bowel obstruction in the neonatal period[42]. The obstruction is due to inspissation of meconium in the distal ileum. In some cases meconium ileus is complicated by volvulus, atresia, or stenosis. Ultrasound is particularly useful in such a neonate with a gasless abdomen.

On ultrasound, dilated fluid filled or meconium filled bowel loops may be imaged. If a mass is palpated and volvulus is suspected, ultrasound may be useful in identifying the mass as bowel loops. Meconium peritonitis may be present and will be discussed below.

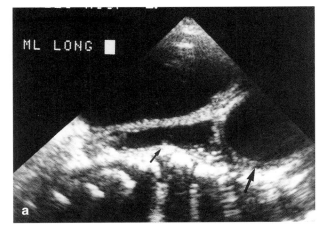

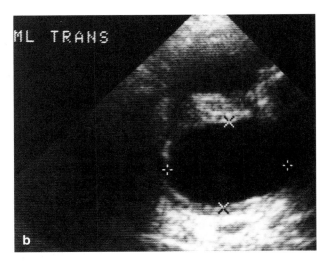

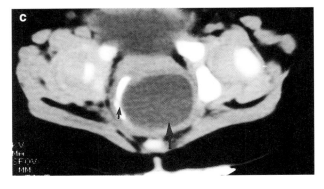

**Figure 9** (**a**) Longitudinal view of the pelvis in an 8-week-old with a rectal duplication cyst. A cystic structure with a well-defined wall is (large arrow) in contact with the rectum (small arrow). (**b**) Transverse view of the cystic mass in the same patient. (**c**) CT of the pelvis following rectal contrast in the same patient. The rectal lumen (small arrow) is displaced laterally by the fluid filled rectal duplication (large arrow)

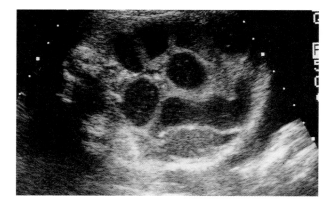

**Figure 10** Prenatal ultrasound demonstrating multiple fluid filled dilated bowel loops in a child found at birth to have ileal atresia

## Meconium peritonitis

Meconium peritonitis results from an *in utero* bowel perforation. It is most commonly associated with bowel atresias. However, it may also be seen in association with meconium ileus, or may be present in an asymptomatic neonate in whom the *in utero* bowel perforation sealed without sequelae[43]. Plain films demonstrate calcific densities scattered throughout the abdomen which are the result of calcified meconium in the peritoneal cavity. In a male infant in whom the processus vaginalis is patent, multiple calcifications may be present in the scrotum. An abnormal gas pattern may be present (Figures 12a,b and 13a,b).

On ultrasound, multiple echogenic foci which shadow are present in the abdomen, representing the calcifications seen on plain film. If there is an accompanying bowel abnormality, dilated fluid filled bowel loops may be seen.

## Colon

### Intussusception

Intussusception is a common problem in children between the ages of 6 months and 2 years and may present with vomiting, intermittent abdominal pain, distension, abdominal mass, and rectal bleeding. Although rare, intussusception has been reported in the neonatal period in full term as well as preterm infants[44,45]. Mortality may be higher in these infants as signs and symptoms are often more difficult to recognize. In contrast to the older infant and child, a lead point is usually present in

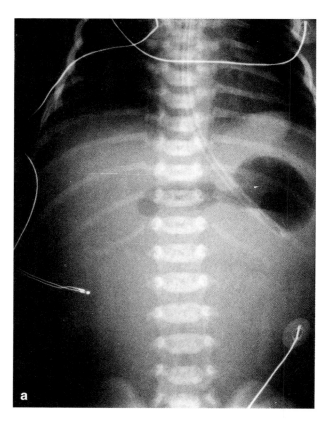

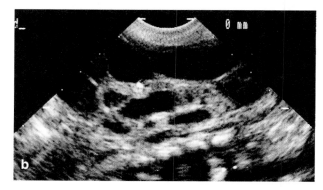

**Figure 11** (a) Supine abdominal radiograph in a newborn male. Air is present in the stomach and proximal duodenum, both of which are displaced superolaterally by an abdominal mass in the mid-abdomen. (b) Longitudinal ultrasound of the abdomen in the same patient. Multiple fluid filled bowel loops are present. At surgery, volvulus with distal small bowel atresia was found

neonates with intussusception. Lead points may include Meckel's diverticula, mesenteric cysts, and duplication cysts[44].

Intussusception has a characteristic appearance on ultrasound[46]. On transverse images, a thick sonolucent ring with a central echogenic area is

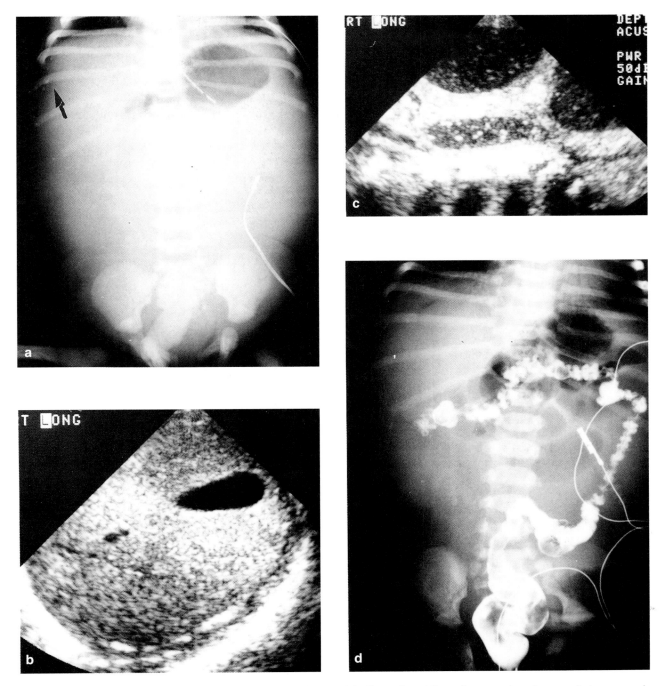

**Figure 12** (**a**) Supine abdominal radiograph in a newborn with distension. There is a paucity of gas and the stomach is displaced superiorly. Calcifications are seen in the right upper quadrant (arrow) consistent with meconium peritonitis. (**b**) Longitudinal ultrasound of the right upper quadrant in the same patient demonstrates highly echogenic foci seen along the periphery of the liver, consistent with meconium peritonitis. (**c**) Longitudinal view of the abdomen demonstrates multiple fluid and debris filled bowel loops in the right lower quadrant. (**d**) Barium enema in the same infant. A microcolon is present

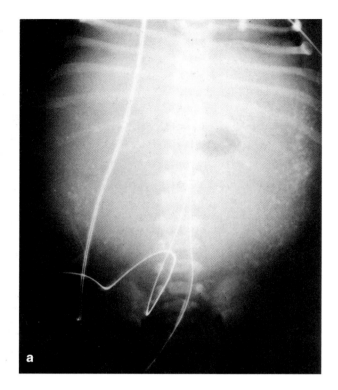

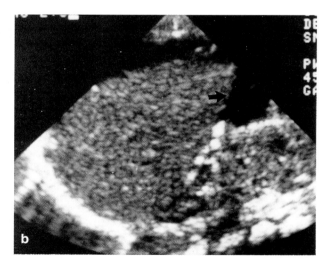

**Figure 13** (**a**) Abdominal radiograph in a newborn with distension. Calcifications, most prominent in the flanks, represent meconium peritonitis. (**b**) Ultrasound in the same patient demonstrates ascites (arrow) and highly echogenic areas consistent with calcifications from meconium peritonitis

seen, termed the 'doughnut sign'. Longitudinally, similar findings have been called the 'pseudo-kidney sign'. The sonolucent ring is believed to represent the edematous infolded loop of the intussusceptum while the echogenic central area

represents its compressed mucosa. Often, concentric rings are present. These result from visualization of additional bowel wall layers within the intussusception (Figure 14a,b). Doppler ultrasound may be able to evaluate vascularity of the intussusception and predict ischemia[47].

Intussusception may be reduced with hydrostatic pressure or by air reduction. Frequently, an edematous ileocecal valve may be seen during fluoroscopy, which may mimic a residual intussusception. Ultrasound may be helpful in distinguishing between persistent intussusception and an edematous ileocecal valve. The edematous valve appears as a small sonolucent rim with an echogenic center. It is distinguishable from intussusception in that its cross-section diameter is smaller than that of an intussusception and it lacks the concentric rings frequently seen in intussusception[48] (Figure 14 c,d).

## Necrotizing enterocolitis

Bowel distension, pneumatosis, and portal venous gas are the hallmark radiographic features of necrotizing enterocolitis (NEC). Pneumatosis and portal venous gas are radiographically evident in 70% and 25% of cases respectively[49]. Neonates may develop clinical signs of NEC and have non-diagnostic radiographs. In this setting, ultrasound may be useful in diagnosing NEC, although ultrasound does not replace the plain radiograph or clinical assessment. Early diagnosis enables aggressive management which decreases morbidity and mortality.

Ultrasound may detect gas in the portal venous system not yet visualized on plain radiographs. Portal venous gas appears as highly echogenic foci moving within the portal venous system or as highly echogenic patches within the hepatic parenchyma[49,50].

Ultrasound may also be useful in detecting bowel wall thickening, intramural gas, and ascites, particularly in the setting of a gasless abdomen[51,52]. These findings, too, may be apparent by ultrasound before plain film detection[52].

## Mesenteric cyst

A benign mesenteric cyst may present as a large intra-abdominal mass in the newborn period. It may be unilocular or septated, and may demonstrate acoustic enhancement. It may be associated

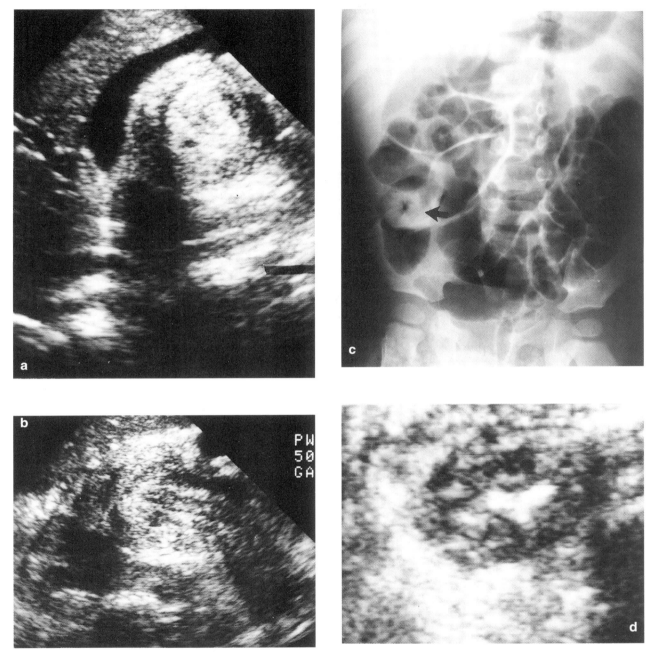

**Figure 14** (**a**) Transverse view of the right flank, demonstrates the 'target sign' of concentric rings of bowel in an intussusception. (**b**) In longitudinal view, the intussusception has the 'pseudokidney' appearance. (**c**) Supine abdominal film in same patient following reduction of intussusception demonstrates a swollen ileocecal valve (arrow). (**d**) Ultrasound of the right lower quadrant following reduction. An echogenic ring is present in the right lower quadrant with an echogenic center. This was smaller in diameter than the intussusception and lacked concentric rings. This represents the swollen ileocecal valve

with congenital abnormalities of the lymphatic system such as lymphangiomas. Differential diagnosis includes duplication cyst and, in a female infant, ovarian cyst presenting as an abdominal mass. Rarely, the walls of mesenteric cysts calcify[53]. The double wall sign is absent in mesenteric cysts, which distinguishes them from enteric duplication cysts[41].

# References

1. Haller JO, Cohen HL. Pediatric ultrasound in the 1990s. *Pediatr Ann* 1992;21:7982–6
2. Hayden CK Jr. Ultrasonography of the gastrointestinal tract in infants and children. *Abdominal Imag* 1996;21:9–20
3. Blumhagen JD. The role of ultrasonography in the evaluation of vomiting in infants. *Pediatr Radiol* 1986;16:267–70
4. Teele RL, Share JC. The abdominal mass in the neonate. *Semin Roentgenol* 1988;23:175–84
5. Siegel MJ. Gastrointestinal tract. In Siegel MJ, ed. *Pediatric Sonography*, 2nd edn. New York: Raven Press, 1995;263–300
6. Swischuk LE, Hayden CK Jr, Fawcett HD, *et al.* Gastroesophageal reflux: how much imaging is required? *Radiographics* 1988;8:1137–45
7. Wright LL, Baker KR, Meny RG. Ultrasound demonstration of gastroesophageal reflux. *J Ultrasound Med* 1988;7:471–5
8. Westra SJ, Wolf BHM, Staalman CR. Ultrasound diagnosis of gastroesophageal reflux and hiatal hernia in infants and young children. *J Clin Ultrasound* 1990;18:477–85
9. O'Keeffe FN, Stansberry SD, Swischuk LE, *et al.* Antropyloric muscle thickness at US in infants: what is normal? *Radiology* 1991;178:827–30
10. Stringer DA, Daneman A, Brunelle F, *et al.* Sonography of the normal and abnormal stomach (excluding hypertrophic pyloric stenosis) in children. *J Ultrasound Med* 1986;5:183–8
11. Katz ME, Blocker SH, McAlister WH. Focal foveolar hyperplasia presenting as an antral-pyloric mass in a young infant. *Pediatr Radiol* 1985;15:136–7
12. McAlister WH, Katz ME, Perlman JM, *et al.* Sonography of focal foveolar hyperplasia causing gastric obstruction in an infant. *Pediatr Radiol* 1988;18:79–81
13. Peled N, Dagan O, Babyn P, *et al.* Gastric-outlet obstruction induced by prostaglandin therapy in neonates. *N Engl J Med* 1992;327:505–10
14. Goodlad RA, Madgwick AJ, Moffat MR, *et al.* Prostaglandins and the gastric epithelium: effects of misoprostol on gastric epithelial cell proliferation in the dog. *Gut* 1989;30:316–21
15. Kessler H, Smulewicz JJ. Microgastria associated with agenesis of the spleen. *Radiology* 1973;107:393–6
16. Hoehner JC, Kimura K, Soper RT. Congenital microgastria. *J Pediatr Surg* 1994;29:1591–3
17. Moulton SL, Bouvet M, Lynch FP. Congenital microgastria in a premature infant. *J Pediatr Surg* 1994;29:1594–5
18. Chew AL, Friedwald JP, Donovan C. Diagnosis of congenital antral web by ultrasound. *Pediatr Radiol* 1992;22:342–3
19. Moccia WA, Astacio JE, Kaude JV. US demonstration of gastric duplication in infancy. *Pediatr Radiol* 1981;11:52–4
20. Herman TE, Oser AB, McAlister WH. Tubular communicating duplications of esophagus and stomach. *Pediatr Radiol* 1991;21:494–6
21. Naik DR, Bolia A, Boon AW. Demonstration of a lactobezoar by ultrasound. *Br J Radiol* 1987;60:506–8
22. Lambrecht L, Robberecht E, Deschynkel K, *et al.* Ultrasound evaluation of gastric clearing in young infants. *Pediatr Radiol* 1988;18:314–18
23. Rollins MD, Shields MD, Quinn RJM, *et al.* Pyloric stenosis: congenital or acquired? *Arch Dis Child* 1989;64:138–47
24. Forman HP, Leonidas JC, Kronfeld GD. A rational approach to the diagnosis of hypertrophic pyloric stenosis: do the results match the claims? *J Pediatr Surg* 1990;25:262–6
25. Stevenson RJ. Non-neonatal intestinal obstruction in children. *Surg Clin North Am* 1985;65:1217–34
26. Stunden RJ, LeQuesne GW, Little KET. The improved ultrasound diagnosis of hypertrophic pyloric stenosis. *Pediatr Radiol* 1986;16:200–5
27. Haller JO, Cohen HL. Hypertrophic pyloric stenosis: diagnosis using US. *Radiology* 1986;161:335–9
28. Swischuk LE, Hayden CK Jr, Stansberry SD. Sonographic pitfalls in imaging of the antropyloric region in infants. *Radiographics* 1989;9:437–47
29. Ball TI, Atkinson GO, Gay BB Jr. Ultrasound diagnosis of hypertrophic pyloric stenosis: real-time application and the demonstration of a new sonographic sign. *Radiology* 1983;147:499–502
30. Cohen HL, Schechter S, Mestel AL, *et al.* Ultrasonic 'double track' sign in hypertrophic pyloric stenosis. *J Ultrasound Med* 1987;6:139–43
31. Spevak MR, Ahmadjian JM, Kleinman PK, *et al.* Sonography of hypertrophic pyloric stenosis: frequency and cause of nonuniform echogenicity of the thickened pyloric muscle. *Am J Radiol* 1992;158:129–32
32. Blumhagen JD, Noble HGS. Muscle thickness in hypertrophic pyloric stenosis: sonographic determination. *Am J Radiol* 1983;140:221–3
33. Blumhagen JD, Maclin L, Krauter D, *et al.* Sonographic diagnosis of hypertrophic pyloric stenosis. *Am J Radiol* 1988;150:1367–70
34. Westra SJ, de Groot CJ, Smits NJ, *et al.* Hypertrophic pyloric stenosis: use of the pyloric volume measurement in early US diagnosis. *Radiology* 1989;172:615–19
35. Pracros JP, Sann L, Genin G, *et al.* Ultrasound diagnosis of midgut volvulus: the 'whirlpool' sign. *Pediatr Radiol* 1992;22:18–20

36. Zerin JM, DiPietro MA. Superior mesenteric vascular anatomy at US in patients with surgically proved malrotation of the midgut. *Radiology* 1992;183:693–4

37. Dufour D, Delaet MH, Dassonville M, *et al*. Midgut malrotation, the reliability of sonographic diagnosis. *Pediatr Radiol* 1992;22:21–3

38. Smet MH, Marchal G, Ceulemans R, *et al*. The solitary hyperdynamic pulsating superior mesenteric artery: an additional dynamic sonographic feature of midgut volvulus. *Pediatr Radiol* 1991;21:156–7

39. Cohen HL, Haller JO, Mestel AL, *et al*. Neonatal duodenum: fluid-aided US examination. *Radiology* 1987;164:805–9

40. Hayden CK, Boulden TF, Swischuk LE, *et al*. Sonographic demonstration of duodenal obstruction with midgut volvulus. *Am J Radiol* 1984;143:9–10

41. Barr LL, Hayden CK Jr, Stansberry SD, *et al*. Enteric duplication cysts in children: are their ultrasonographic wall characteristics diagnostic? *Pediatr Radiol* 1990;20:326–8

42. Leonidas JC, Berdon W. The neonate and young infant. In Silverman FN, Kuhn JP, eds. *Caffey's Pediatric X-ray Diagnosis*. 9th edn. St. Louis, MO: Mosby, 1993:2059–62

43. Estroff JA, Bromley B, Benacerraf BR. Fetal meconium peritonitis without sequelae. *Pediatr Radiol* 1992;22:277–8

44. Patriquin HB, Afshani E, Effman E, *et al*. Neonatal intussusception. Report of 12 cases. *Radiology* 1977;125:463–6

45. Price KJ, Roberton NRC, Pearse RG. Intussusception in preterm infants. *Arch Dis Child* 1993;68:41–2

46. Swischuk LE, Hayden CK, Boulden T. Intussusception: indications for ultrasonography and an explanation of the doughnut and pseudokidney signs. *Pediatr Radiol* 1985;15:388–91

47. Lam AH, Firman K. Value of sonography including color Doppler in the diagnosis and management of longstanding intussusception. *Pediatr Radiol* 1992;22:112–14

48. Rohrschneider W, Troger J, Betsch B. The postreduction donut sign. *Pediatr Radiol* 1994;24:156–60

49. Lindley S, Mollitt DL, Seibert JJ, *et al*. Portal vein ultrasonography in the early diagnosis of necrotizing enterocolitis. *J Pediatr Surg* 1986;21:530–2

50. Robberecht EA, Afschrift M, De Bel CE, *et al*. Sonographic demonstration of portal venous gas in necrotizing enterocolitis. *Eur J Pediatr* 1988;147:192–4

51. Weinberg B, Peralta VE, Diakoumakis EE, *et al*. Sonographic findings in necrotizing enterocolitis with paucity of abdominal gas as the initial symptom. *Mt Sinai J Med* 1989;56:330–3

52. Morrison SC, Jacobson JM. The radiology of necrotizing enterocolitis. *Clin Perinatol* 1994;21:347–63

53. Geer LL, Mittelstaedt CA, Staab EV, *et al*. Mesenteric cyst: sonographic appearance with CT correlation. *Pediatr Radiol* 1984;14:102–4

# Sonographic evaluation of the neonatal biliary system

5

*Rona J. Orentlicher and Jack O. Haller*

Over the last several years, marked improvements have been made in the field of ultrasound. With the advances made in color Doppler imaging and the use of high frequency transducers, the detection of biliary disease has improved considerably.

## Technique

Ultrasound evaluation of the biliary system is ideally performed on a patient who has fasted for 8 to 12 hours, a difficult task in a neonate. Images are obtained in both longitudinal and transverse projections and the neonate is studied in the supine position. To detect movement in the gall-bladder lumen, additional positions can be obtained such as a decubitus or upright position. A complete examination of the biliary system includes evaluation of the liver, gallbladder, and pancreas as well as visualization of the common bile duct (CBD) and its branches. To help differentiate the CBD from adjacent vascular structures, color Doppler can be a very useful tool.

## The normal biliary system

While there have been many studies documenting normal adult ultrasound measurements, few studies have been reported describing the normal pediatric, and in particular, neonatal gallbladder and biliary system. However, normal parameters of the gallbladder in children can be significant, since often the only sign of disease is gallbladder distention and wall thickening[1].

The gallbladder shape is important. The gallbladder should be elliptical in shape and demonstrate an anechoic lumen on ultrasound. In assessing gallbladder size and length, McGahan *et al.* found there was a gradual increase with age[1]. The gallbladder had a mean length of 2.5 cm from birth to one year of age, increasing to approximately 6 cm at 12–16 years. The gallbladder lumen diameter was approximately 1 cm at one year and

2 cm at 12–16 years. Wall thickness was fairly constant at less than 3 mm throughout childhood. Hernanz-Schulman *et al.* performed a prospective study that documented the size of the CBD increasing slowly and linearly with age[2]. The caliber of the pediatric CBD was significantly different from that of healthy adults. The common bile duct of neonates was found to be 1.6 mm or less in inner-wall to inner-wall diameter increasing to 2.5–3 mm in childhood and early adolescence. Carroll *et al.* documented similar results, with a width of greater than 2 mm – highly suspicious for biliary pathology[3].

## Anomalies

During routine ultrasound evaluation of the biliary tract and, in particular, the gallbladder, it is not uncommon to find a wide assortment of anomalies. Anomalies of the gallbladder can be categorized based on location, number, and shape[4].

The gallbladder is normally located in the inferior aspect of the liver in the region of the interlobar fissure. Anomalies in gallbladder location are rare. They include intrahepatic, retro-peritoneal, retrohepatic, and left-sided positioning both with and without situs inversus. Therefore, if the gallbladder is not located in its normal position during sonography, care must be taken to rule out an ectopic location.

An absent gallbladder is rare. Other unusual anomalies in number include a bifid or duplicated gallbladder. These can be well demonstrated using ultrasound.

The gallbladder is usually oval; however, common variations in shape can occur. In particular, the junctional fold, which is the gallbladder body folded on the infudibulum and the phrygian cap, which is the gallbladder fundus folded on the body[5] (Figure 1). True septated gallbladders are rare; however, this anomaly has been reported to predispose to stasis and possible infection[4,6,7] (Figure 2).

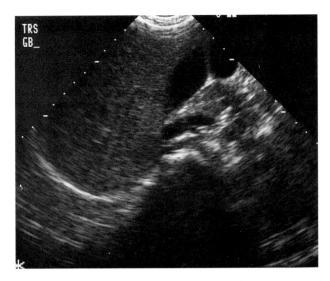

**Figure 1** Junctional fold. Sonogram of the right upper quadrant shows an apparent septation in the region of the gallbladder that resulted from the gallbladder folding on itself

## The enlarged gallbladder

The number of reported neonatal cases of gallbladder enlargement in the past few years have increased significantly, particularly in premature infants. Several terms have been used in the literature to describe gallbladder enlargement. These terms include 'gallbladder distention'[8], 'hydrops'[9,10], 'acute dilation'[11]; and 'acalculous cholecystitis'[12]. The distinction by ultrasound between a normally distended gallbladder and pathologic gallbladder enlargement can often be difficult. If there is also evidence of cystic duct obstruction, a pathologic cause for the enlargement is more likely. For our discussion, we will reserve the term 'acalculous cholecystitis' for true gallbladder inflammation with its other associated findings such as a thick wall, stone formation and dilated CBD. This abnormality may require possible surgical intervention. The terms hydrops, acute dilation and gallbladder distention will be used for non-inflammatory enlargement often requiring medical intervention only and will be discussed in further detail below.

There are several causes of gallbladder enlargement in the neonate (Table 1). One of the most common causes of gallbladder enlargement is the use of total parenteral nutrition (TPN). The mechanism by which TPN causes gallbladder enlargement is based on biliary physiology. The flow of bile is controlled by the sphincter of Oddi. During interdigestive periods, the sphincter is

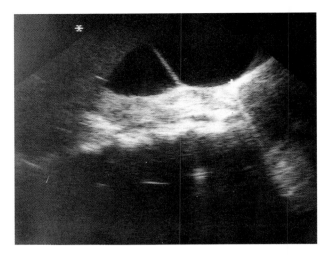

**Figure 2** Septated gallbladder. Longitudinal section of the right upper quadrant shows a gallbladder with a true septation within it dividing the gallbladder into two compartments

**Table 1** Causes of enlarged gallbladder in neonates

| |
| --- |
| Sepsis |
| Total parenteral nutrition or starvation |
| Dehydration |
| Nodes |
| Congenital anomalies |
| Stones |
| Hepatitis |
| Burns |
| Trauma |

closed and bile accumulates in the gallbladder. During periods of active digestion, the gallbladder contracts by neural and hormonal stimulation, there is sphincter relaxation, and bile is emptied from the gallbladder. TPN and starvation inhibit the neural and hormonal stimulation, thereby resulting in the accumulation of large amounts of bile in the gallbladder leading to significant enlargement[13,14].

Another cause of gallbladder enlargement is sepsis, a common etiology in premature infants. The gallbladder distention may be secondary to cystic duct obstruction from surrounding edema, adenopathy, or it may be the result of biliary atony similar to a dynamic ileus of the intestines from a similar cause[8,15].

Neonatal gallbladder enlargement secondary to obstruction can lead to true cholecystitis. The obstruction may be caused by a congenital anomaly of the biliary or cystic ducts leading to stone formation or anomalies caused by the small bowel such as a duodenal web[8,12]. Secondary obstruction, such as from adjacent lymphadenopathy, can develop from a wide variety of causes, such as hepatitis, leptospirosis, or upper respiratory infections.

Gastroenteritis can lead to dehydration, biliary stasis, and ultimately gallbladder enlargement. Several infectious agents, such as bacterial or parasitic have been reported to directly involve the gallbladder leading to distention[12,16,17] (Table 2).

## Acute cholecystitis

Acute cholecystitis in infants is a relatively rare disease and, unlike adults, is often an acalculous cholecystitis. In adults and in older children, the classic triad of upper right quadrant pain, vomiting and fever is very helpful to the clinician and the radiologist in localizing the problem to the gallbladder and biliary system. In neonates, the clinical presentation is often more confusing and, given that cholecystitis is relatively rare, often overlooked as the source of the problem.

Ultrasound should be the initial screening test in any infant suspected of cholecystitis. It permits rapid evaluation of the gallbladder and biliary system as well as the ability to assess the surrounding structures such as the liver and pancreas for other disease processes[18].

There are several sonographic signs of cholecystitis that have been discussed in the literature and are similar to adults (Table 3).

As previously discussed, an infant gallbladder wall is considered thick if it measures greater than 3 mm in diameter. A layer of sonolucency in the thickened wall may represent localized edema and/or necrosis[18]. Although in the past an isolated ultrasound finding of a thickened gallbladder wall was considered strong evidence for the diagnosis of cholecystitis, recent literature has described this finding in other conditions (Figure 3). These include hypoalbuminemia (possibly causing accumulation of fluid within the wall), ascites (causing a halo effect from free intraperitoneal fluid), a recent meal (physiologic thickening from a contracted wall), or poor systemic venous drainage with secondary venous hypertension[19].

A hyper-reflective gallbladder wall is another sign of disease. It is felt to represent fibrosis, is associated with stagnant bile or sludge, and is often seen in chronic cholecystitis. On ultrasound, sludge is seen as non-shadowing, low level echoes within the gallbladder lumen that often move slowly with changes in position. Identifying sludge

**Table 2**   Infectious organisms causing distention

*Salmonella typhi*
*Escherichia coli*
*Vibrio cholera*
*Ascaris lumbricoide*
*Giardia lamblia*
*Leptospirosis*
*Pseudomonas*
*Serratia marcescens*
*Streptococcus viridans*
*Staphylococcus aureus*
*Clostridium welchii*

**Table 3**   Ultrasound signs of cholecystitis

Thick wall > 3 mm (67% sensitivity)
Halo sign
Hyper-reflective wall
Sludge
Stones
Murphy's sign
Dilated common bile duct

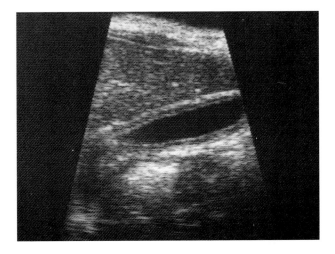

**Figure 3**   Thick walled gallbladder. The sonogram of the gallbladder shows a thick wall composed of an echogenic inner wall, hypoechoic middle wall and an echogenic outer wall. This has been known as a striped or halo effect and was originally thought to be specific for cholecystitis

on ultrasound should prompt the examiner to look for signs of gallbladder wall thickening since sludge may represent cystic duct obstruction from inflammation or calculi[18].

Failure to visualize the gallbladder on ultrasound is another possible sign of disease, therefore, the gallbladder fossa should be carefully evaluated. If the gallbladder is not visualized, either the patient has not fasted for long enough or the gallbladder is diseased. A repeat ultrasound can be obtained after proper fasting or a nuclear medicine scan can be obtained to confirm the gallbladder location[18].

Although rare in infants, complications of cholecystitis include empyema, pericholecystic abscess, and perforation. As described by Kane, the ultrasonographic signs of empyema consist of medium-to-coarse intraluminal echoes within the gallbladder which do not layer or cause acoustic shadowing[20]. These echoes are felt to represent purulent, fibrinous debris as well as focal exudate within the gallbladder. The lack of layering is due to the increased viscosity of the bile[20]. Perforation of the gallbladder is usually due to an area of wall gangrene or infarction. Sonographic signs include biliary ascites, symbolizing an acute process; a distinct pericholecystic fluid collection or abscess, often seen in a subacute process; or a biliary fistula seen in a chronic perforation. The gallbladder wall is often thickened and indistinct and cholelithiasis is often present. The diagnosis is best made with an accompanying hepatobiliary radionuclide study. On the nuclear medicine study, a distinct rim of radionuclide can be seen in the pericholecystic region or with biliary ascites; there is a band of radionuclide around the periphery of the abdomen with a photopenic center[21].

## The jaundiced infant

During the first weeks of life, the majority of healthy infants may experience transient jaundice. Benign causes lead to increased unconjugated (indirect) bilirubin and follow a self-limiting course. Possible etiologies include breastfeeding or the mobilization of sequestered blood from a large cephalohematoma. An increased conjugated (direct) bilirubin level is never benign. For infants with conjugated hyperbilirubinemia, evaluation should be undertaken for anatomic, infectious, or metabolic causes of the cholestasis.

Of the many causes of conjugated hyperbilirubinemia, approximately 60–80% are caused by neonatal hepatitis, biliary atresia, and choledochal cyst. An algorithm is recommended in these cases of neonatal jaundice. The diagnostic approach should begin with laboratory testing to rule out most non-anatomical diseases. If the lab tests are not diagnostic, ultrasound is the next step to rule out any structural abnormalities such as choledochal cyst, bile duct stricture, or biliary stones. If ultrasound is not diagnostic, then

scintigraphy with iminodiacetic acid should be performed.

The ultrasound findings in neonatal hepatitis are non-specific. The liver echogenicity is normal and the liver size is normal or increased. The intra- and extrahepatic ducts are also normal in caliber. The gallbladder may be enlarged, normal, or not well visualized. Hepatobiliary scintigraphy after pretreatment with phenobarbitol will demonstrate normal hepatic uptake with delayed excretion into the gastrointestinal tract. With severe hepatitis, hepatic uptake is decreased.

Biliary atresia is, pathologically, periportal fibrosis with intrahepatic small duct proliferation and focal or total absence of extrahepatic ducts. The ultrasound findings in biliary atresia are generally non-specific. The liver is usually normal in size and echogenicity. Bile duct dilatation does not occur despite distal obstruction since the intra- and extrahepatic ducts are diseased and contracted. The gallbladder is small or absent. Utilizing hepatic scintigraphy, the liver has normal or decreased uptake and excretion, with absent tracer activity into the gastrointestinal tract. Therefore, isotope excretion into the duodenum proves biliary patency and eliminates biliary atresia as a possible diagnosis. Conversely, absence of duodenal uptake even with good hepatic uptake may represent biliary atresia but does not rule out other intrahepatic disorders[22].

## Gallstones

Although often regarded as a disease of adults, cholelithiasis is becoming a common entity in children, in particular, infants and adolescents. Most often seen in children with various hereditary blood dyscrasias, gallstones can develop secondary to many causes (Table 4).

Approximately 80% of all gallstones contain cholesterol as the chief component. Usually the gallstones are mixed, containing other elements such as calcium carbonate, phosphate, or bilirubinate. Pigmented black stones are composed of less than 25% cholesterol and contain different concentrations of calcium carbonate, bilirubinate, or phosphate. These pigmented stones are seen in the hemolytic anemias. Brown pigmented stones also contain calcium bilirubinate as their chief component, but are also composed of calcium palmitate and cholesterol. They develop in cases of Caroli's disease, strictures, and sclerosing cholangitis. Brown pigmented stones are virtually 100% radiolucent, while 50–60% of black stones are

**Table 4** Risk factors associated with cholelithiasis

Idiopathic[23]
Total parenteral nutrition[24]
Gallbladder atony – stasis – infection (systemic)[25]
Dehydration–vomiting[25]
RDS–BPD–furosemide–sepsis[23]
Gallbladder and bile duct anomalies[26]
Morphine usage in mother[27]
Bowel resection – NEC – Volvulus[28]

RDS, respiratory distress syndrome; BPD, bronchopulmonary dysplasia; NEC, necrotizing enterocolitis

radio-opaque and 15% of cholesterol stones are radio-opaque. Gallstones in infants and neonates are most commonly pigmented, composed of calcium bilirubinate with smaller amounts of calcium carbonate and phosphate.

The pathophysiology of stone formation varies with the predisposing disease but three possible mechanisms appear to predominate: (1) decreased concentration of bile salts secondary to impaired enterohepatic circulation, (2) increased deposition of unconjugated bilirubin, and (3) stasis.

The development of cholesterol is dependent on the local concentration of cholesterol in bile. Cholesterol is normally insoluble in aqueous solution but is maintained in solution by bile salts. Therefore, high levels of cholesterol or low levels of bile salts predispose to stone formation. Bile salts normally enter the digestive system, are reabsorbed and accumulate in the liver by way of the enterohepatic circulation. In cases where the enterohepatic circulation is impaired, such as necrotizing enterocolitis (NEC) or bowel resection, the low levels of bile salts lead to stone formation.

Increased deposition of unconjugated bilirubin is due to increased secretion by the liver from excessive breakdown of hemoglobin. This occurs in various hemolytic anemias leading to the common side-effect of stone disease.

Another factor involved in stone formation in children is impaired gallbladder function. The gallbladder normally responds to cholecystokinin (CCK), which is stimulated by oral feedings, by contracting and emptying its contents. CCK also initiates increased fluid secretion in the gallbladder and causes relaxation of the sphincter of Oddi leading to gallbladder dilution and emptying into the small intestine. Lack of food (from vomiting, TPN, or starvation) leads to decreased CCK stimulation and gallbladder stasis. Morphine usage in the mother has been reported to decrease gastrointestinal motility in neonates and, therefore, decrease of CCK release. Morphine can also lead

to gallbladder hypotonicity resulting in sludge formation and subsequent gallstones[27].

One of the most common causes for the increased incidence of gallstones in premature infants, aside from improved ultrasound technique, is the increased use of TPN. TPN-induced cholestasis was initially described by Peden *et al.* in 1971[29]. As discussed above, one possible mechanism is lack of CCK stimulation and resulting stasis. Other possible hypotheses include an immature hepatocellular enzyme system with resultant disturbance in conjugated bilirubin transport which ultimately impairs bile secretion. An abnormality in amino acid metabolism that impairs bile salt formation has also been implicated in TPN-induced stone formation[24].

Ultrasound is a very sensitive method for detection of gallstones. Gallstones are highly echogenic, intraluminal gallbladder masses with posterior shadowing. The diagnosis can be made with confidence if the echogenic mass demonstrates mobility with a change in patient position. On occasion, the stone is not mobile if it is impacted in the gallbladder neck or is adherent to the gallbladder wall. Very small stones may not demonstrate posterior shadowing. If stones are suspected in such cases, it is advantageous to change the patient's position, since small stones piled on top of each other may elicit enough of a posterior shadow to confirm the diagnosis. Differentiating tumefactive sludge or sludge balls from small stones can be difficult sonographically since sludge is echogenic material with no posterior shadowing.

Prenatal gallstone formation is not common; it has been reported in approximately six cases. With increasing use of obstetrical ultrasound and more sophisticated equipment, gallstones may be seen with more frequency. The gallbladder on a fetal ultrasound can be identified in the right upper quadrant as an ovoid fluid-filled structure. Care must be taken not to confuse the gallbladder with a vascular structure, in particular, the umbilical vein. Use of Doppler can differentiate gallbladder from adjacent vascularity (Figure 4). In several of the reported cases of fetal gallstones, acoustic shadowing was not well demonstrated. This may be due to the small size of the stones or may mean that the stones were actually echogenic sludge[30–32] (Figure 5).

Aside from one documented case of mild 'spherocytosis' in a newborn with documented fetal gallstones other abnormalities have not been reported. There have been no reported cases of gallstones leading to any symptoms, and most have resolved spontaneously. Therefore, surgical or

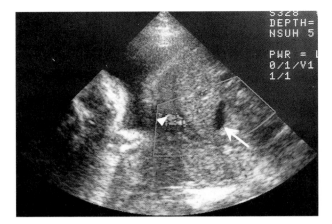

**Figure 4** Fetal gallbladder. Scan of the fetal abdomen shows the gallbladder (arrow) and the adjacent Doppler effect from the umbilical vein (v)

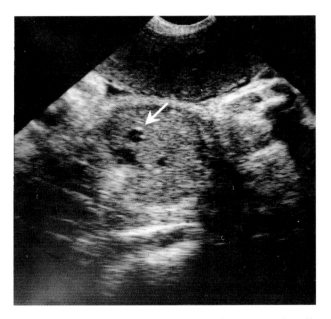

**Figure 5** Fetal gallstone. Scan of the neonatal gallbladder shows an echogenic foci in the fetal gallbladder (arrow) consistent with a fetal gallstone. The mother had no predisposing factors

other intervention is not warranted. However, close monitoring for any biliary structural abnormalities, such as a choledochal cyst, is warranted. Evaluation for any inherited hemolytic anemia or blood group incompatibility is also indicated. We recommend a more careful assessment of the gallbladder and surrounding structures after delivery and follow-up ultrasounds to document resolution of the gallstones, usually within six months. If gallstones persist after 12 months, or if there are symptoms, many advise

cholecystectomy to prevent complications such as biliary obstruction, pancreatitis, perforation with bile peritonitis or sepsis. Others take a more conservative approach[23,28,30,32–35].

The simultaneous development of nephrolithiasis and cholelithiasis has been reported in only a few cases. The reported cases were in premature infants, weighing less than 1500 grams, who have bronchopulmonary dysplasia (BPD), and received furosemide and total parenteral nutrition (TPN) therapy. With removal of the furosemide, the renal stones often disappeared; however, the gallstones were more likely to remain[36] (Figure 6).

## Choledocholithiasis

Common bile duct stones in infancy are unusual. In one large series, common duct stones were reported in 6–21% of children with cholelithiasis[37]. Although CBD stones may originate from the gallbladder, 'primary' CBD stones, originating in the intra- or extrahepatic ducts, can occur. Possible etiologies include inspissated bile plug, biliary atresia, neonatal hepatitis, and choledochal cysts. CBD stones have been implicated in the formation of obstructive hepatic damage, perforation, and pancreatitis[37,38].

Ultrasound can be a useful tool in documenting common bile duct stones (Figure 7). The diagnosis can be made with dilatation of the bile ducts and the presence of echogenic material commonly located in the distal duct, just above the sphincter. Ultrasound, however, can often be limited by overlying bowel gas in infants, contributing to the reported 20–60% CBD stone detection success rate.

## Bile plug syndrome

This rare entity, first described in 1969 by Bernstein, represents a mechanical obstruction of the CBD by a plug of secretions and bile. The mechanism is unclear. It was first reported in infants with maternal Rh and ABO blood group incompatibility, complicated by hemolysis with subsequent obstruction of the CBD by inspissated sludge. With early detection and exchange transfusions, perinatal hemolysis is now a rare cause of bile plug syndrome. Causative factors now include TPN use, prematurity, dehydration, infection, and intestinal abnormalities[38,39].

While the plugs commonly resolve spontaneously, they have been known to cause cholangitis. Any sign of infection or biliary dilatation is considered

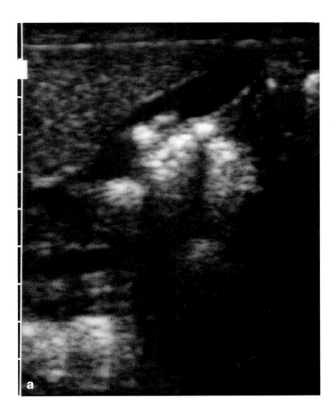

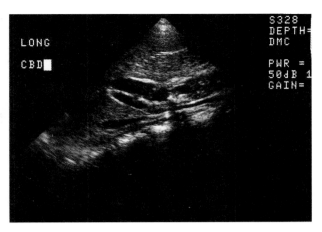

**Figure 7** Choledocholithiasis. Scan of the right upper quadrant in the region of the common bile duct shows dilatation of the common bile duct with an echogenic focus with shadowing at the distal portion

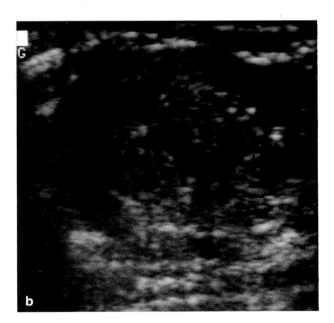

**Figure 6** Simultaneous fetal renal and gallbladder stones. (**a**) Longitudinal scan of the gallbladder shows echogenic foci in the gallbladder that layered when the baby was placed in an erect position. These were consistent with gallstones. (**b**) Scan of the right kidney shows echogenic material in the inferior portions of each pyramid some of which shadowed. The child had been getting furosemide and total parenteral nutrition

indication for prompt diagnosis and treatment. The diagnosis can be made with a liver biopsy. With asymptomatic jaundiced infants, ultrasound monitoring for evidence of biliary dilatation is warranted. Frank choledochal obstruction remains a surgical disease. Treatment options for the biliary obstruction include mucolytic agents to dissolve the concretions, saline irrigation of the biliary tree, choledochotomy, sphincterotomy, and in more severe cases biliary–enteric anastomoses[37–40].

## Choledochal cyst

Cystic dilatation of the biliary system, also known as choledochal cyst, is relatively rare in the United States. The disorder appears to be more common in Asia, as evidenced by the large amount of Japanese literature on the subject. There are no familial reports or studies implicating genetic factors[41]. It is generally considered a disorder of infancy and children, although there have been cases reported of patients ranging in age from newborn to 80 years old. Sixty per cent of cases are diagnosed in patients less than 10 years of age[42–44].

The prevalence of choledochal cysts is higher in females, at a ratio of approximately 4:1. The classic triad of pain, abdominal mass, and jaundice is seen in only a minority of patients. In the young infant, the most likely presentation is one of intermittent jaundice and abdominal mass. In older children and adults, the presentation is more likely fever, vomiting, jaundice, and abdominal pain, possibly related to complications from pancreatitis and cholangitis[42].

The classification of choledochal cysts is complicated, possibly due to an increasing attempt to include all forms of bile duct dilatation under the umbrella of choledochal cyst[43–46] (Figure 8). Type I cysts are the most common, accounting for 80–90% of cases. Type I is a dilatation of a portion of the CBD and is often associated with proximal and/or distal atresia or obstruction. Type I is further subdivided based on the shape of the involved dilatation. Type IA involves a dilatation of the CBD with marked dilatation of all or part of the extrahepatic ducts. Type IB consists of a focal, segmental dilatation of the CBD, usually involving the distal CBD. Type II cyst is a diverticulum of the CBD. Type III cyst is a choledochocele that involves only the intraduodenal portion of the CBD. Type III is the rarest type and felt by some to be a separate entity from a choledochal cyst[46–48]. Type IV is dilatation of the intrahepatic and extrahepatic ducts. Type V, also known as Caroli's disease, involves dilatation of intrahepatic ducts.

The pathogenesis of choledochal cysts remains controversial. Early theories have included faulty epithelial proliferation and recanalization of the embryonic CBD, vascular accidents, and intrauterine rupture of the bile duct. Other groups theorized that the origin of the cyst was due to a combination of weakening of the CBD wall in a specific segment and increased intraductal pressure from a distal obstruction[44,45,49–51].

In 1974, Landing hypothesized that neonatal hepatitis, biliary atresia, and choledochal cysts represented manifestations of 'infantile obstructive cholangiopathy'. He theorized that a virus caused scarring of the biliary ducts resulting in sclerosis, obstruction, and biliary cyst formation[52].

In 1973, Babbitt et al. hypothesized an anomalous arrangement of the pancreaticobiliary ductal system. The anomaly is a failure of normal separation of the pancreatic and common bile ducts. The result is that the distal CBD enters the duct of Wirsung at a right angle approximately 2 to 3.5 cm from the ampulla of Vater, a far more proximal insertion than the normal anatomy. The resultant reflux of pancreatic juices into the biliary tree causes cholangitis with inflammation, scarring, and eventual biliary dilatation[53,54]. Many clinical investigators have subsequently concurred with Babbitt's hypothesis[55,56].

By contrast, other investigators dispute that the anomalous pancreaticobiliary union is the sole etiology for choledochal cyst formation. Some feel this etiology pertains to the cyst that forms in older children and adults and helps to explain the classic triad of mass, jaundice, and pain. However, in

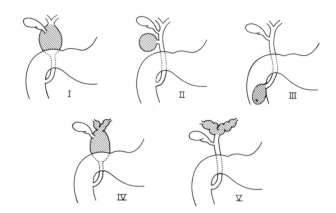

**Figure 8** Diagrammatic representation of the five types of choledochal cysts. See text for descriptions

neonates, where the common presentation is jaundice and acholic stool, an inherent weakness in the CBD wall with associated distal obstruction is a more likely etiology. This theory would also explain the high association of neonatal choledochal cyst with biliary atresia[57,58].

In the past, barium studies were used to document choledochal cysts. There was displacement of the stomach and duodenum with a widening of the duodenal C-loop. A more definitive diagnosis can now be made with the advent of ultrasound, hepatobiliary scintigraphy, and computed tomography (CT). Ultrasound is the best initial study in any patient with jaundice. Sonography can demonstrate a cystic mass in the porta hepatis that is contiguous with the bile duct, separate from the gallbladder, with possible intra- and/or extrahepatic ductal dilatation. CT is often more sensitive in documenting intrahepatic dilatation and in assessing the distal CBD which may be obscured on ultrasound by bowel gas. Nuclear medicine studies document that the cystic structure seen on ultrasound or CT communicates with the biliary system and determines the presence of distal obstruction. In the older patients with a nonobstructed choledochal cyst, a filling defect is seen in the porta hepatis which gradually fills in on delayed images, indicating a communication with the biliary system[5,42].

The most common complication of a choledochal cyst is stones in the gallbladder, within the cyst (Figure 9), or in the intrahepatic or pancreatic duct. Other more detrimental complications include cirrhosis with portal hypertension, cholangitis, and pancreatitis. For these reasons, rapid treatment is essential. A liver biopsy should be performed to determine the prognosis. The preferred surgical management is cyst excision with a Roux-en-Y hepaticoenterostomy. CBD and gallbladder carcinoma have also been associated with choledochal cysts. Long term follow-up is indicated since excision of the cyst does not preclude the possibility of carcinoma developing in the intrahepatic ducts. Definitive treatment for a choledochocele is transduodenal marsupialization[42–44,59,60].

## Caroli's disease

In 1958, Jacques Caroli first described this condition, communicating cavernous ectasia of the intrahepatic ducts, as an uncommon cause of chronic hepatobiliary disease[61,62]. Congenital biliary dilatation is common in Japan but uncommon in the West. The disorder is felt to be autosomal recessive, although it has been reported in families[63]. The etiology of congenital biliary dilatation is still not clear but is similar to the choledochal cyst. Some possible mechanisms include neonatal occlusion of the hepatic artery causing biliary ischemia and dilatation or a developmental defect in the supportive structure of the duct wall[62,64]. There is still ongoing debate as to whether Caroli's disease is a separate entity from a choledochal cyst or part of a continuing spectrum.

The disorder is becoming more and more common in children. Two forms of the disorder have been described. The rare pure form (Type I) is characterized by saccular intrahepatic biliary dilatation, originally described by Caroli, and the more common form (Type II) is associated with congenital hepatic fibrosis. Type I usually presents with fever and abdominal pain due to stone formation, cholangitis, or hepatic abscess formation. The cause of death is due to septicemia or hepatic abscess. Type II presents with signs and symptoms related to hepatic fibrosis and portal hypertension such as varices and gastrointestinal hemorrhage. Biliary stones and cholangitis are usually absent in Type II disease. Death from Type II disease is commonly from portal hypertension or liver failure[62]. Caroli's disease is associated with other entities such as recessive polycystic kidney disease, choledochal cyst, medullary sponge kidney, and cholangiocarcinoma[65].

Ultrasound is an excellent method for evaluating Caroli's disease. In the Type I form, ultrasound will demonstrate saccular intrahepatic anechoic spaces converging toward the porta hepatis. Communication between the sacculi and bile ducts is important in making the diagnosis. A

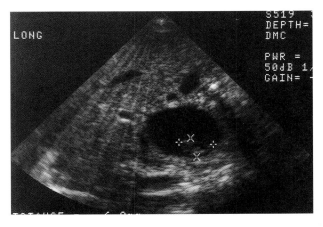

**Figure 9**  Choledochal cyst. A scan of the right upper quadrant shows a cystic mass in the inferior aspect of the liver which contains echogenic debris (Xs). Upon removal a choledochal cyst was confirmed

clue to the diagnosis is fibrovascular bundles that contain a portal vein and a hepatic artery that bridge the sacculi. The fibrovascular bundle may protrude into the dilated duct and appear on ultrasound as a linear bridge or central dot. Doppler can be helpful in demonstrating vascularity in the bundle. In the Type II form, associated with hepatic fibrosis, the ultrasound findings correspond to the underlying fibrotic liver disease. These findings include a shrunken echogenic liver, splenomegaly, ascites, and varices. Stones are almost always absent[62]. The ultrasound study can be limited in the evaluation of Caroli's disease, particularly in visualizing the peripheral and common bile ducts. Overlying bowel gas can obscure the image. For further evaluation, CT or cholangiogram is recommended.

## Spontaneous perforation of the common bile duct

Although spontaneous perforation of the CBD is relatively rare, it is the second most common cause of surgical jaundice in the neonate, second only to biliary atresia. Most cases of perforation have similar clinical history, radiographic results, and operative findings to suggest the diagnosis. The perforation occurs almost exclusively in neonates. It is most common between the first and third months of life. The patient presents with ascites, mild jaundice, and acholic stool. Scrotal and inguinal swellings secondary to bilious ascites pressure have also been described. Bile peritonitis is usually aseptic, unless ascending cholangitis develops, leading to spillage of infected bile through the perforation[66,67]. The liver function tests are usually normal except for an elevated bilirubin: an important laboratory distinction from neonatal hepatitis.

The pathogenesis of spontaneous perforation of the CBD is still not clear. Distal CBD obstruction secondary to stenosis or stones has been implicated. However, it is unclear as to whether the stones are the cause or the result of the perforation. Bile stones and sludge may form in a temporarily dysfunctional CBD distal to a perforation. Another more attractive hypothesis is an area of CBD wall weakness due to a localized embryologic mural malformation. The location of the perforation is very commonly the anterior wall of the CBD at its insertion into the cystic duct, suggesting that this area is particularly vulnerable to developmental abnormalities. An area of weakness may be due to pancreatic juice reflux from an anomaly of the pancreaticoduodenal junction, similar to choledochal cyst formation, or from bile duct ischemia. The main arterial supply to the CBD is located on either side of and posterior to the CBD, making the anterior wall vulnerable to impaired blood supply. Increased biliary pressures from stone or sludge formation can thus result in dilatation of the CBD wall and perforation[67,68].

Ultrasound findings of ascites, with or without loculated fluid and normal intra- and extrahepatic ducts suggest the diagnosis[66] (Figure 10a). The loculated fluid, often located in the porta hepatis, can form a pseudocyst composed of inflammatory tissue. A radioisotope scan confirms the diagnosis by demonstrating the extravasated marker free in the peritoneal cavity. Radioisotope may also accumulate in the pseudocyst[68] (Figure 10b).

Treatment usually consists of intraoperative drainage with spontaneous closure and subsequent cure. Care must be taken not to confuse the inflammatory pseudocyst and ascites with a ruptured choledochal cyst. An erroneous surgical anastomosis to the flimsy sac can have disastrous results. The combination of ultrasound, nuclear medicine, and clinical findings should lead to the correct preoperative diagnosis.

## Trauma to the biliary system

Ultrasound is not considered the ideal initial modality in studying patients with suspected liver, biliary, or splenic injuries. Ultrasound can miss significant trauma due to increased overlying

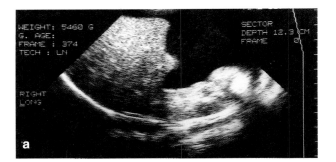

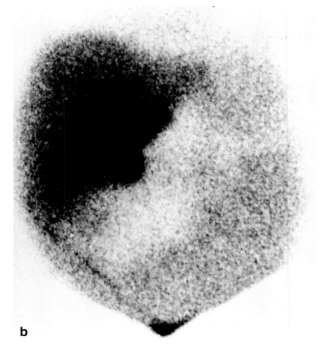

**Figure 10** (a) Longitudinal scan of the right upper quadrant shows an apparently normal liver with ascites in the more caudal portion of the abdomen. (b) Hida scan of the abdomen shows significant radionuclide activity dispersed throughout the abdomen. There is a halo effect. There is also increased accumulation of radioisotope in the region of the porta hepatis. At surgery a loculated biloma in the porta hepatis was found as well as free bile peritonitis

bowel gas, and poorly visualize the entire liver and spleen, particularly at the dome of the diaphragms. CT is considered far more sensitive in detecting traumatic injury in children. Ultrasound, however, can be used successfully to non-invasively follow already diagnosed injuries once the exact location has been defined. In addition, ultrasound can demonstrate ascites, pseudocysts, bilomas, and hemobilia. Color Doppler has not been fully explored in evaluating hepatobiliary trauma but may eventually play a secondary role in the diagnostic workup of pediatric trauma.

Perforation of the biliary system secondary to trauma is a rare occurrence. When it occurs it can produce free leakage of bile into the peritoneal cavity. A biloma can form if the leaking bile is encapsulated[69]. The diagnosis is suggested on ultrasound by a large anechoic mass, although differentiation from a hematoma is usually not possible. The confirmation of a bile leak is best demonstrated with nuclear medicine, when radioisotope collects in the bile leak or biloma.

## Syndromes of the biliary system

There are five major syndromes associated with the biliary system: Alagille syndrome, asplenia syndrome, polysplenia syndrome, Bardet–Biedle syndrome, and Caroli's syndrome.

Alagille syndrome (arteriohepatic dysplasia) is an autosomal disease associated with intrahepatic bile duct hypoplasia. Other clinical manifestations include unusual facial characteristics such as a broad forehead, widely spaced eyes, and underdeveloped mandible; ocular and cardiovascular abnormalities (usually peripheral stenosis, sometimes tetralogy of Fallot); vertebral arch defects and tubulointerstitial nephropathy. Mental retardation is sometimes present[70]. Ultrasound is generally non-specific in diagnosing the syndrome, although the liver has been reported to be echogenic.

Asplenia syndrome (Ivemark syndrome), also called bilateral lung right-sidedness, can be transmitted in either an autosomal recessive or dominant mode. The syndrome is associated with agenesis or malpositioning of the gallbladder and a centrally located liver. Other manifestations include cardiac, gastrointestinal and genitourinary anomalies. There are bilateral trilobed lungs and eparterial bronchi.

Polysplenia syndrome, also called bilateral lung left-sidedness, can present in infancy or adulthood. The biliary abnormalities include extrahepatic biliary atresia, absent gallbladder, and a pre-duodenal portal vein. Other manifestations, aside from multiple spleens, include azygos continuation of the IVC, bowel malrotation, situs inversus, and preduodenal portal vein. If liver transplant is considered for biliary atresia, careful assessment of the hepatic vascular anatomy is necessary.

Bardet–Biedle syndrome has an autosomal recessive transmission and is associated with pigmentary retinal degeneration, obesity, polydactyly, genital hypoplasia, and mental retardation. Cystic dilatation of the intrahepatic and common bile duct is a less common manifestation.

# References

1. McGahan JP, Phillips HE, Cox KL. Sonography of the normal pediatric gallbladder and biliary tract. *Radiology* 1982;144:355–7
2. Hernanz-Schulman M, Ambrosino MM, Freeman PC, *et al.* Common bile duct in children: sonographic dimensions. *Radiology* 1995;195:193–5
3. Carroll BA, Oppenheimer DA, Muller HH. High frequency real time ultrasound of the neonatal biliary system. *Radiology* 1982;145:437–40
4. Meilstrup JW, Hopper KD, Thieme GA. Imaging of gallbladder variants. *Am J Radiol* 1991;157:1205–8
5. Rumack CM, Wilson SR, Charboneau JW. *Diagnostic Ultrasound*, 5th edn. St. Louis: Mosby-Yearbook, 1991;108:135–6, 1168
6. Adear H, Barki Y. Multiseptate gallbladder in a child: incidental diagnosis on sonography. *Pediatr Radiol* 1990;20:192
7. Simon M, Tandon BN. Multiseptate gallbladder: a case report. *Am J Roentol* 1963;80:84–6
8. Peevy KJ, Weissman HJ. Gallbladder distention in septic neonates. *Arch Dis Child* 1982;57:75–6
9. Robinson AE, Erwin JH, Wiseman HJ, *et al.* Cholecystitis and hydrops of the gallbladder in the newborn. *Radiology* 1977;122:749–51
10. Goldthorn JF, Thomas DW, Ramos AD. Hydrops of the gallbladder in stressed premature infants. *Clin Res (A)* 1980;28:122–3
11. Bowen A. Acute gallbladder dilatation in a neonate: emphasis on ultrasonography. *J Pediatr Gastroenterol Nutr* 1984;3:304–5
12. Dewan PA, Stokes KB, Solomon JR. Pediatric acalculous cholecystitis. *Pediatr Surg Int* 1987;2:120–1
13. Banfield WF. Physiology of the gallbladder. *Gastroenterology* 1975;69:770–7
14. Barth RA, Brasch RC, Filly RA. Abdominal pseudotumor in childhood: distended gallbladder with parenteral nutrition. *Am J Radiol* 1981;136:341–3
15. El Shafie M, Mah CL. Transient gallbladder distention in sick premature infants: the value of ultrasonography and radionuclide scintigraphy. *Pediatr Radiol* 1986;16:468–71
16. Cohen EK, Stringer DA, Smith CR, *et al.* Hydrops of the gallbladder in typhoid fever as demonstrated by sonography. *J Clin Ultrasound* 1986;14:633–5

17. Roca M, Sellier N, Mensire A, *et al*. Acute acalculous cholecystitis in Salmonella infection. *Pediatr Radiol* 1988;18:421–3

18. Greenberg M, Kangarloo H, Sachiko TC, *et al*. The ultrasonographic diagnosis of cholecystitis and cholelithiasis in children. *Radiology* 1980;137: 745–9

19. Patriquin HB, DiPietro M, Barber FE, *et al*. Sonography of thickened gallbladder wall: causes in children. *Am J Radiol* 1983;141:57–60

20. Kane RA. Ultrasonographic diagnosis of gangrenous cholecystitis and empyema of the gallbladder. *Radiology* 1980;134:191–4

21. Bergman AB, Neiman HL, Kraut B. Ultrasonographic evaluation of pericholecystic abscess. *Am J Radiol* 1979;132:201–3

22. Kirks DR, Coleman RE, Filston HC, *et al*. An imaging approach to persistent neonatal jaundice. *Am J Radiol* 1984;142:461–5

23. Holcomb GW Jr, Holcomb GW III. Cholelithiasis in infants, children and adolescents. *Pediatr Rev* 1990; 2:268–75

24. Callahan J, Haller JO, Cacciarelli AA, *et al*. Cholelithiasis in infants: association with total parenteral nutrition and furosemide. *Radiology* 1982;143:437–9

25. Cheng ERY, Okoye MI. Cholecystitis and cholelithiasis in children and adolescents. *J Nat Med Assoc* 1986;78:1073–8

26. Kassner EG, Klotz DH. Cholecystitis and calculi in a diverticulum of the gallbladder. *J Pediatr Surg* 1975; 10:967–8

27. Figueroa-Colon RF, Tolaymat N, Kao JCS. Gallbladder sludge and lithiasis in an infant born to a morphine user mother. *J Pediatr Gastroenterol Nutr* 1990;10:234–8

28. Williams HJ, Johnson KW. Cholelithiasis: a complication of cardiac valve surgery in children. *Pediatr Radiol* 1984;14:146–7

29. Peden V, Witzleben C, Skelton M. Total parenteral nutrition. *J Pediatr* 1971;78:180–1

30. Abitt PL, McIlhenny J. Prenatal detection of gallstones. *J Clin Ultrasound* 1990;18:20

31. Beretsky I, Lankin D. Diagnosis of fetal cholelithiasis using real-time high resolution imaging employing digital detection. *J Ultrasound Med* 1983;2:381–3

32. Klingensmith WC, Cioffi-Ragan DT. Fetal gallstones. *Radiology* 1988;167:143–4

33. Keller MS, Markle BM, Laffey PA, *et al*. Spontaneous resolution of cholelithiasis in infants. *Radiology* 1985;157:345–8

34. Schirmer WJ, Grisoni ER, Gauderer MWL. The spectrum of cholelithiasis in the first year of life. *J Pediatr Surg* 1989;24:1064–7

35. Takiff H, Fonkalsrud EW. Gallbladder disease in childhood. *Am J Dis Child* 1984;138:565–8

36. Ramey SL, Williams JL. Nephrolithiasis and cholelithiasis in a premature infant. *J Clin Ultrasound* 1986;14:203–6

37. Lilly JR. Common bile duct calculi in infants and children. *J Pediatr Surg* 1980;15:577–80

38. Pariente D, Bernard O, Gauthier F, *et al*. Radiologic treatment of common bile duct lithiasis in infancy. *Pediatr Radiol* 1989;19:104–7

39. Brown DM. Bile plug syndrome: successful management with a mucolytic agent. *J Pediatr Surg* 1990;25:351–2

40. Jonas A, Yahav A, Fradkin A, *et al*. Choledocholithiasis in infants: diagnostic and therapeutic problems. *J Pediatr Gastroenterol Nutr* 1990;11:513–7

41. O'Neill JA, Templeton JM, Schnaufer L, *et al*. Recent experience with choledochal cyst. *Ann Surg* 1987;5: 533–40

42. Kim OH, Chung HJ, Choi BG. Imaging of the choledochal cyst. *Radiographics* 1995;15:69–88

43. Todani T, Watanabe Y, Narusue M, *et al*. Congenital bile duct cysts. *Am J Surg* 1977;134:263–9

44. Yamaguchi M. Congenital choledochal cyst. *Am J Surg* 1980;140:653–7

45. Alonzo-Lej F, Rever WB, Pessagno DJ. Congenital choledochal cyst: with a report of 2 patients and an analysis of 94 cases. *Int Abst Surg* 1959;108:1–30

46. Swischuk LE. *Imaging of the Newborn, Infant, and Young Child*. 3rd edn. Baltimore, MD: Williams & Wilkins 1989:520–1

47. Wearn FG, Wiot JF. Choledochocele: not a form of choledochal cyst. *J Can Assoc Radiologists* 1982;33: 110–12

48. Kangaloo H, Sarti DA, Sample WF, *et al*. Ultrasonographic spectrum of choledochal cysts in children. *Pediatr Radiol* 1980;9:15–8

49. Saito S, Ishida M. Congenital choledochal cyst (cystic dilatation of the common bile duct). *Prog Pediatr Surg* 1974;6:63–90

50. Crittenden SL, McKinley MJ. Choledochal cyst: clinical features and classification. *Am J Gastroenterol* 1985;80:643–7

51. Yotsuyanagi S. Contributions to etiology and pathology of idiopathic cystic dilatation of the common bile duct with report of three cases. *Gann* 1936;30:601–752

52. Landing BH. Consideration of the pathogenesis of neonatal hepatitis, biliary atresia and choledochal cyst – the concept of infantile obstructive cholangiopathy. *Prog Pediatr Surg* 1974;5:113–39

53. Babbitt DP, Starshak RJ, Clemett AR. choledochal cyst: a concept of etiology. *Am J Radiol* 1973;119:57–62

54. Howell CG, Templeton JM, Weiner S, *et al*. Antenatal diagnosis and early surgery for choledochal cyst. *J Pediatr Surg* 1983;18:387–93

55. Kato T, Hebiguchi T, Matsuda K, *et al*. Action of pancreatic juice on the bile duct: pathogenesis of congenital choledochal cyst. *J Pediatr Surg* 1981; 16:146–51

56. Jona JZ, Babbitt DP, Srashak RJ, *et al*. Anatomic observations of etiologic and surgical considerations in choledochal cyst. *J Pediatr Surg* 1979;14:315–20

57. Lilly JR. Surgery of coexisting biliary malformations in choledochal cyst. *J Pediatr Surg* 1979;14:643–7

58. Torrisi JT, Haller JO, Velcek FT. Choledochal cyst and biliary atresia in the neonate. *Am J Radiol* 1990;155:1273–6

59. Ozawa K, Yamada T, Matsumoto Y, *et al*. Carcinoma arising in a choledochocele. *Cancer* 1980;45:195–7

60. Manning PB, Polley TZ Jr, Oldham KT. Choledochocele: an unusual form of choledochal cyst. *Pediatr Surg Int* 1990;5:22–6

61. Caroli J, Couinaud C. Une affection nouvelle sans doute congenitale, desvoies biliares: la dilatation kystique unilobaire des canaux hepatiques. *Semin Hop Paris* 1958;34:496–502

62. Miller WJ, Sechtin AG, Campbell WL, *et al*. Imaging findings in Caroli's disease. *Am J Radiol* 1995; 165:333–7

63. Iwafucai M, Ohsawa Y, Naito S, *et al*. Familial occurrence of congenital bile duct dilatation. *J Pediatr Surg* 1990;11:513–7

64. Mittelstaedt CA, Volberg FM, Fischer GJ, *et al*. Caroli's disease: sonographic findings. *Am J Radiol* 1980;134:585–7

65. Takehara Y, Motoichiro T, Masaaki N, *et al*. Caroli's disease associated with polycystic kidney: its noninvasive diagnosis. *Radiat Med* 1989;7:13–5

66. Fawcett HD, Hayden CK, Swischuk LE, *et al*. Spontaneous extrahepatic biliary duct perforation in infancy. *J Can Assoc Radiol* 1986;37:206–7

67. Lilly JR, Weintraub WH, Altman RP. Spontaneous perforation of the extrahepatic bile ducts and bile peritonitis in infancy. *Surgery* 1974;75:664–73

68. Lloyd DA, Mickel RE. Spontaneous perforation of the extra-hepatic bile ducts in neonates and infants. *Br J Surg* 1980;67:621–3

69. Gould L, Patel A. Ultrasound detection of extrahepatic encapsulated bile: 'biloma'. *Am J Radiol* 1979;132:1014–5

70. Nelson WE. *Textbook of Pediatrics*, 13th edn. Philadelphia: WB Saunders, 1987:831

# The neonatal adrenal gland

*John C. Leonidas and Sudha P. Singh*

## 6

## Normal anatomy

The adrenal glands are retroperitoneal structures, sitting on the anteriomedial aspect of the upper pole of each kidney. They are composed of the cortex, of mesodermal origin, which consists of three layers (zona glomerulosa, zona fasciculata and zona reticularis), and the medulla, of neuroectodermal origin, which is enveloped by the cortex. The fetal adrenal gland is enlarged because of a markedly thickened cortical layer, the fetal cortex, which is covered by a thin layer of what will eventually become the cortex in the adult. Soon after birth the fetal cortex begins to involute. Mineralocorticoids (including aldosterone) are being secreted by cells of the zona glomerulosa. Cells in the zona fasciculata and reticularis secrete glucocorticoids and sex hormones, whereas adrenalin and noradrenalin are being produced by the cells of the medulla under the influence of sympathetic preganglionic fibers. Because of their size the neonatal adrenal glands are very easily visualized by ultrasound (US). On longitudinal scans they appear as V or Y shaped structures composed of a hyperechoic inner layer, representing the medulla, and a hypoechoic outer cortex (Figure 1). On transverse scans the glands have an elongated elliptical shape, with a more or less linear inner hyperechoic layer (medulla) surrounded by the hypoechoic cortex (Figure 2).

The length of the neonatal glands, measured on longitudinal scans along the axis of the longest limb, has been determined to range from 0.9 to 3.6 cm. The thickness or width of each limb has been found to be from 0.2 to 0.5 cm[1,2].

## Congenital adrenal hyperplasia

Congenital adrenal hyperplasia (CAH) or adrenogenital syndrome has an incidence between 1 : 7000 and 1 : 10 000[3]. It is the most common cause of female pseudohermaphroditism (46XX with normal female internal genitalia but virilization of the external genitalia). Although the syndrome can result from an adrenal adenoma, most often it results from simple hyperplasia in the neonatal age group. In male infants adrenal hyperplasia is more difficult to detect. It is caused by deficiency of one of the enzymes involved in adrenal steroid metabolism, C-21 hydroxylase deficiency being the most common[3]. Each deficiency is transmitted as an autosomal recessive

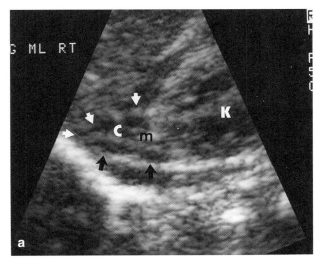

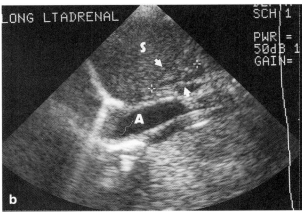

**Figure 1** (a) Longitudinal scan of the right adrenal gland shows the triangular V shaped gland outlined by arrows. Note the echogenic medulla (m) surrounded by the hypoechoic cortex (C). K, right kidney. (b) Longitudinal view of the left adrenal gland (between cursors and arrows). A, aorta; S, spleen

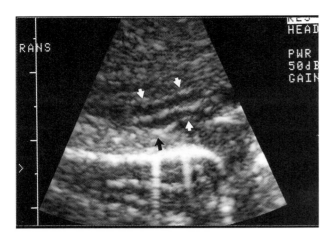

**Figure 2** Transverse view of the right adrenal gland (arrows). Note the centrally located echogenic medulla enveloped by the hypoechoic cortex

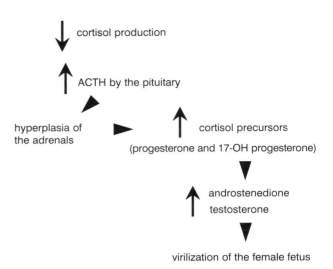

**Figure 3** Diagram of the chemical events leading to virilization in congenital adrenal hyperplasia. ACTH, adrenocorticotrophic hormone

trait (Figure 3). Thirty per cent of these patients have a concomitant mineralocorticoid (aldosterone) insufficiency leading to salt loss. High progesterone and 17-OH progesterone enhance this effect by competing for the aldosterone receptors.

CAH is the most common cause of ambiguous genitalia in females while males typically present with a salt-losing crisis in the first 1–2 weeks of life or precocious puberty later in childhood. The degree of virilization is determined by the stage of intrauterine life at which the genitalia are subjected to excess androgens[4]. If the onset is before the 12th week of intrauterine life, there is retention of the urogenital sinus and labio-scrotal fusion with urethral extension on to the genital tubercle. If the onset is after the 12th week of intrauterine life, only clitoral hypertrophy and labial scrotalization may be seen. Normal female internal genitalia develop irrespective of the stage at which the fetus is exposed to increased androgens, because the internal genitalia develop along female lines unless fetal testicular tissue is present.

It is extremely important that the diagnosis be made early because treatment with cortisone stops excessive androgen production and allows normal sexual development to proceed. Biochemical confirmation of diagnosis may require days. This causes delay in diagnosis and subsequent onset of therapy.

Sonography is a useful tool at this stage and its role is twofold. It can help make a presumptive diagnosis by demonstrating bilaterally enlarged adrenal glands and by visualizing the internal genitalia can help assign the correct sex at an early stage.

## Sonographic findings

A wrinkled surface of enlarged adrenal glands simulating the cerebriform pattern of the brain gyri with preservation of the normal cortico-medullary differentiation is proposed as a specific pattern to the disease[5] (Figure 4). The pattern is more easily demonstrated with high frequency transducers. Symmetrically enlarged glands with a mean length measurement of 20 mm or greater and mean width measurements of 4 mm or greater suggest the diagnosis[4,6]. However, normal sized adrenals do not preclude a diagnosis of CAH. Another pitfall is the physiologically enlarged neonatal adrenal glands.

## Adrenal hemorrhage

Adrenal hemorrhage occurs almost exclusively in newborns. The exact etiology is still questionable although hypoxia (antenatal, labor-induced or neonatal) is usually associated with this event, and is considered a likely cause. Hypoxia results in reflex shunting of blood away from the splanchnic and visceral vascular bed to preserve circulation to the vital structures, such as the heart and the brain. The ensuing ischemia may cause hemorrhagic infarction of the adrenals[7].

It almost always presents in the first week of life although presentation at 3–4 weeks of age has been reported. It may rarely occur *in utero*, although prenatal detection is indeed uncommon. It occurs on the right side 70% of times and may be

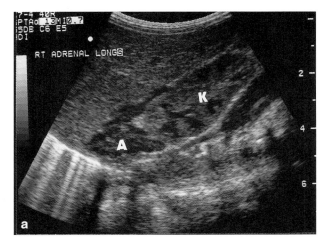

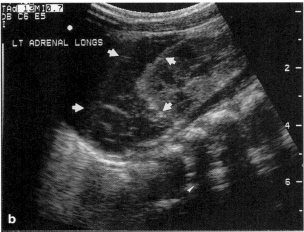

**Figure 4** Bilateral adrenal enlargement of a female newborn with entirely male-appearing external genitalia. (**a**) The right adrenal gland is enlarged, with the largest limb approximately 3.8 cm in length and a width of 1.0 cm of the posterior limb. K, right kidney (**b**) Longitudinal view of the left adrenal. The markedly enlarged gland (arrows) presents a 'cerebriform appearance', with the longest upper limb measuring 4.5 cm and a width of 1.5 cm. A, adrenal

bilateral in 10% of cases[8]. It may involve the whole gland or could be focal. The predisposing factors include obstetrical or birth trauma; maternal diabetes; neonatal sepsis; neonatal hypoxia; and coagulation defects.

The newborn generally presents with anemia and jaundice, often associated with a palpable suprarenal mass displacing the ipsilateral kidney caudally. Renal vein thrombosis, a common association may, however, lead to true renal enlargement. Signs of acute shock may be seen with severe blood loss. Adrenal hemorrhage is most often a self-limited process, and proper conservative management generally results in an uneventful recovery of almost all patients[8]. Adrenal insufficiency is a rare complication of bilateral adrenal hemorrhage.

### Sonographic findings

Ultrasonography is now the mainstay of diagnosis and follow-up of these patients, largely having replaced intravenous pyelography (IVP). The sonographic diagnosis is based upon the chronological changes seen in the echogenicity and size of the lesion. To begin with, adrenal hemorrhage appears as a solid or almost entirely solid lesion obliterating the Y or inverted V appearance of the normal adrenal gland. It may compress or displace the upper pole of the ipsilateral kidney. As liquefaction and necrosis ensue, it acquires a mixed or complex mass pattern and ultimately becomes anechoic and cyst like[8] (Figure 5). The lesion may again become echogenic with posterior acoustic shadowing as dystrophic calcification develops. The rate at which these changes progress varies from patient to patient, and it also depends on the size of the hemorrhage[7].

If the changes in echotexture and a decrease in the size of the lesion are not seen with time, an alternative diagnosis of neonatal neuroblastoma (solid or cystic), adrenal abscess, cortical renal cyst or an obstructed upper excretory tract in a duplicated kidney should be considered. Magnetic resonance imaging (MRI) is useful in defining the mass as being hemorrhagic, but is of limited value as neuroblastoma, the main diagnostic concern, may also be hemorrhagic (Figure 6). Change therefore remains the final diagnostic criterion.

### Inflammatory diseases

Inflammatory diseases of the adrenal glands occur very rarely in the newborn. Adrenal abscesses have been described, either following hematogenous bacterial seeding or complicating adrenal hemorrhage[9]. Plain film radiography and IVP show nonspecific mass effect on the ipsilateral kidney. US demonstrates a hypoechoic cystic mass, occasionally with low level echoes from debris. At times the mass may be complex, depending on the degree of liquefaction of the inflammatory process.

### Adrenal cysts

Adrenal cysts are very rare in the newborn, with the exception of those resulting from hemorrhage. It has been recognized recently however that large

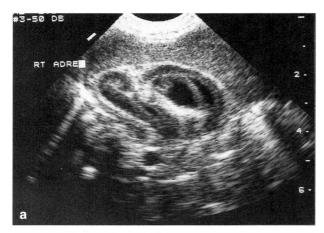

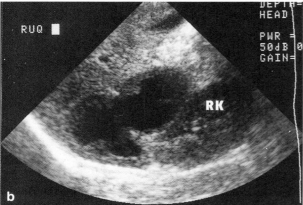

**Figure 5**  (**a**) Right adrenal hemorrhage. Disorganized adrenal pattern, along with a complex mass occupying the central portion of the adrenal. (**b**) Approximately one week later there is expansion of cystic component as the clot continues to liquefy. RK, right kidney

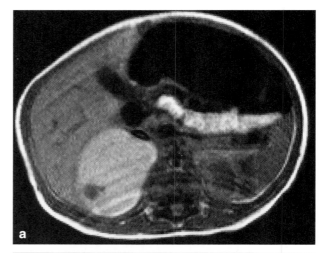

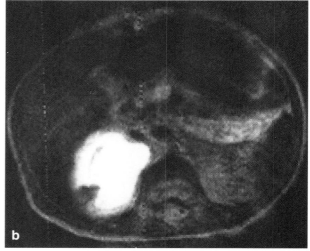

**Figure 6**  Neonatal adrenal hemorrhage. (**a**) T$^1$ weighted MRI shows relatively high signal intensity of the right adrenal mass. (**b**) On this T$^2$ weighted image the adrenal mass becomes even brighter, as expected with a relatively old hemorrhage. Low signal intensity nodule may represent early calcification or hemosiderin deposition

adrenal cysts, most likely developing in pre-existing microcysts, occur in the Beckwith–Wiedemann syndrome. The cysts are unilateral, may become very large and are occasionally filled with blood[10]. Patients with the Beckwith–Wiedemann syndrome are at high risk for the development of Wilms' tumor, hepatoblastoma, gonadoblastoma and adrenocortical carcinoma.

## Wolman disease

Wolman disease is characterized by extensive visceral deposition of cholesterol and triglycerides, caused by a deficiency of lysosomal acid esterase. Cholesterol esters and triglycerides accumulate in the liver, spleen, lungs, adrenals, bone marrow, and gastrointestinal tract, causing a rapidly progressive clinical illness marked by hepato-splenomegaly, vomiting, diarrhea, steatorrhea,

abdominal distention, and adrenal calcification. Death usually occurs during the first six months of life, although there is clinical variability with some cases occurring beyond the neonatal period and characterized by a more protracted course. The disease most often occurs among Iranian Jews, and is probably transmitted as an autosomal recessive metabolic disorder. Pathologically the adrenals are enlarged and contain large histiocytes with coarsely vacuolated cytoplasm. The vacuoles show the histochemical features of cholesterol. There is also extensive calcification of both adrenal glands[11-13]. Both plain film radiographs and IVP show bilateral adrenal calcification. US shows large adrenal glands which are hyperechoic with intense acoustic shadowing consistent with calcification (Figure 7). The degree of calcification of the adrenal glands is most dramatic on computed tomography (CT) scans (Figure 7). Although adrenal calcification may be seen also following simple adrenal hemorrhage, the accompanying severe constitutional symptoms of Wolman disease are very useful in establishing the correct diagnosis.

## Neuroblastoma

Neuroblastoma is the most common solid tumor in infants and children, excluding intracranial tumors, accounting for 7% of all childhood malignancies[14]. Its origin is the primitive neural crest cells, which normally mature into the adrenal medulla and sympathetic ganglia. Neuroblastoma is the least differentiated and therefore most malignant tumor of neural crest origin, whereas the fully differentiated ganglioneuroma represents its mature and benign counterpart in the spectrum of neural crest tumors. An intermediate form of tumor, which is incompletely differentiated, is the ganglioneuroblastoma[1,14].

It is possible that foci of neuroblastoma exist in many otherwise healthy neonates which subsequently mature, never giving rise to malignant disease. Indeed 'neuroblastoma in situ' is a common finding in routine autopsies of newborns and young infants, with an almost 400-fold increase in incidence compared with the overall clinical frequency of neuroblastoma[14]. Conditions associated with a slightly increased incidence of neuroblastoma include neurofibromatosis, neurocristopathy[15], family history of pheochromocytoma, fetal hydantoin and fetal alcohol syndrome, and nesidioblastosis[14]. The peak incidence of neuroblastoma is about 2 years of age, with more than half being younger than 2 years at the time of diagnosis. Occasionally neuroblastoma occurs in the fetus and is fully developed at the time of birth, including metastases to the placenta[14,16].

The abdomen is the site of origin in about two-thirds of cases, and two-thirds of the intra-abdominal tumors originate from the adrenal medulla[1]. Pathologically, neuroblastoma is a solid, nodular mass, with a peripheral rim of cortex and various degrees of necrosis, hemorrhage, and calcification.

Histologically the tumor is composed of small, round, dark staining cells, which in a typical case are arranged in rosette formation. The diagnosis is confirmed by histologic evidence of elements of neural origin or differentiation; at times it is

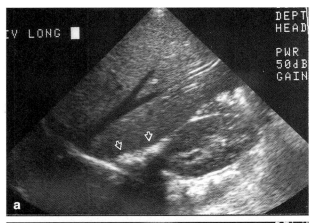

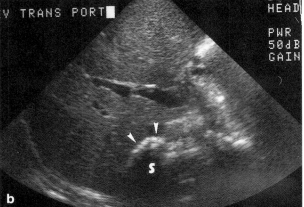

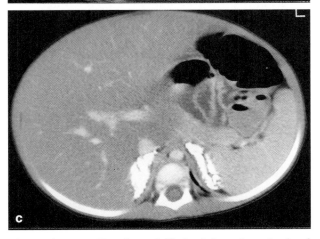

**Figure 7** (a) Heavily calcified right adrenal gland (arrows) with intense acoustic shadowing in an infant with Wolman disease. (b) Transverse image showing calcified gland with acoustic shadowing (S). (c) CT scan in the same infant showing heavily calcified adrenal glands

difficult to differentiate neuroblastoma from other small, round, blue staining cells.

Neuroblastoma tends to metastasize to regional lymph nodes, liver, skeleton, bone marrow, orbits, dura, pleura, and skin. Unlike Wilms' tumor, which is generally confined to the kidney at the time of diagnosis, neuroblastoma is already metastatic (stage IV) at presentation in over one-half of patients[1,14]. There are several staging systems for neuroblastoma. Detailed description of these staging systems is beyond the scope of this chapter. Basically, tumor confined to the site of origin and completely removed is stage I; tumor extending beyond the site of origin, incompletely resected but not crossing the midline is stage II; tumor crossing the midline is stage III; and disseminated tumor is stage IV. Staging however is not the only crucial prognostic factor.

Young age and extra-abdominal site of neuroblastoma are favorable prognostic factors; neonatal neuroblastoma tends to have an exceedingly mild course, even in the presence of metastases at the time of diagnosis (but with metastases limited to the liver, skin or bone marrow, or a combination of these sites). To emphasize the benign course of neuroblastoma in young infants with metastatic disease to the above sites, this group of patients, who would have been technically stage IV, had to be separated and designated as stage IVS. The histology of the tumor, n-myc gene amplification and a host of other clinical, biochemical, and immunologic factors greatly affect prognosis[14].

The most common presenting sign of neuroblastoma is that of an abdominal mass, often with manifestations referred to a metastatic site, such as exophthalmos. In the newborn specifically, the tumor may have been detected on prenatal ultrasound[16]. Physical examination may or may not detect an abdominal mass, depending on the size of the tumor. There is often hepatomegaly, occasionally extreme to the point of causing respiratory distress. In some instances neonates present with hydrops fetalis, with signs of congestive heart failure, ascites, and disseminated intravascular coagulation[14,16]. Acute myoclonic encephalopathy with opsoclonus, presumably of paraneoplastic origin, or diarrhea mimicking gastroenteritis due to increased catecholamine secretion are unusual manifestations of neuroblastoma.

## Imaging of neuroblastoma

This includes plain film radiography, intravenous urography, intravenous pyelography (IVP), US, CT, MRI and nuclear scintigraphy. Plain film radiography is useful in demonstrating a mass effect, hepatomegaly, and especially detection of calcification, which if present increases the likelihood of neuroblastoma substantially. Intravenous urography is performed very rarely

today. Adrenal neuroblastomas cause inferior displacement and usually compression of the upper pole of the kidney, without the effect on the intrinsic architecture of the collecting system seen with intrarenal masses. Sonographic examination shows an adrenal mass compressing and inferiorly displacing the ipsilateral kidney (Figure 8). The tumor is predominantly solid, but with areas of variable echodensities depending on the presence of intratumorous hemorrhage and necrosis. Very bright echodense areas with acoustic shadowing indicate calcification, although most often calcification is fine and punctate and not easily detectable by US. Extra-adrenal neuroblastomas tend to also displace the kidney laterally, are often midline in location and tend to encase the retroperitoneal vessels, including the aorta and inferior vena cava (IVC) with stretching of the renal, celiac, and mesenteric arteries and the renal, splenic, and mesenteric veins. Adrenal neuroblastomas, if large, may displace the IVC, but do not invade it, as often occurs with Wilms' tumor. Occasionally large adrenal masses may also displace the aorta and its branches, and elevate or compress the liver anteriorly if the tumor arises from the right adrenal. The pancreas may be displaced and lifted if the origin is the left adrenal gland. Liver metastases may also be detected; they are most often hypoechoic, although echodensity may vary, and at times only diffuse hepatomegaly is present. Aggressive tumors may invade the kidney, in which case differential diagnosis from Wilms' tumor may be very difficult or impossible.

CT is generally necessary for a more global view of the chest and abdomen, and is more likely to detect calcification (present in over 50% of cases) and liver metastases[16]. MRI seems to offer even better imaging advantages compared with US and CT, by virtue of its multiplanar capability (shared with US), signal characteristics which make liver metastases more obvious (Figure 9) and possible extension into the spinal canal through the intervertebral foramina. The latter is more common with extra-adrenal retroperitoneal neuroblastomas. Nuclear scintigraphy with bone scanning agents (Tc99m MDP) is needed for detection of bone metastases. Demonstration of the primary tumor is also common, as in most cases there is tumor uptake of bone-seeking radionuclides. Metaiodobenzylguanidine (MIBG) or somatostatin analog scanning is promising for tumor detection, although results today are mixed regarding the sensitivity of these agents. Despite some limitations US is readily available, quickly performed, and without the need for sedation. It

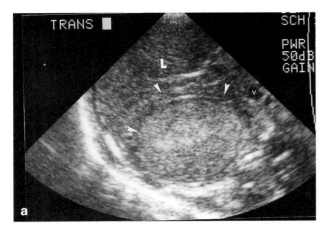

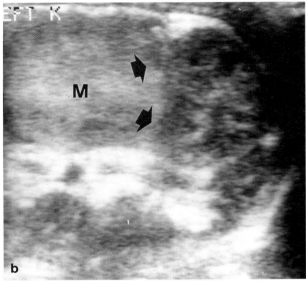

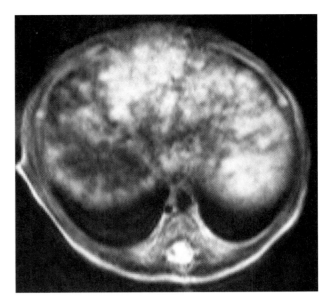

**Figure 9**  T² weighted MRI in a newborn with neuroblastoma metastatic to the liver. Note diffuse high signal intensity nodules almost replacing the enlarged liver. These nodules were not recognized on US or CT

**Figure 8**  (**a**) Neonatal adrenal neuroblastoma presenting as an incidental solid adrenal mass (arrows) which had been seen initially *in utero*. L, liver. (**b**) In another neonate this left neuroblastoma indents and displaces the left kidney (arrows). M, mass

gives good information regarding the location and extent of the tumor, its relationship to vessels and nodal involvement. MRI and nuclear scintigraphy may offer needed supplementary information. It has been suggested that the variable echotexture of neuroblastoma compared with the more homogenous appearance of Wilms' (albeit with scattered cystic areas seen often in the latter) may be useful in differential diagnosis, when the exact origin of the mass (extrarenal *vs.* intrarenal) is not obvious, or when one is dealing with an intrarenal neuroblastoma[17].

Another difficulty in the differential diagnosis of neuroblastoma in the newborn is posed by its similarities with neonatal adrenal hemorrhage. Adrenal hemorrhage may appear solid early on,

and neuroblastoma may undergo hemorrhage and appear cystic. *In utero* neuroblastoma generally appears as a solid mass. Adrenal hemorrhage is very rare on prenatal US[18], so that the mere presence of an adrenal mass *in utero* strongly favors neuroblastoma. On postnatal sonography the best feature is the presence or absence of change. Adrenal hemorrhage rapidly evolves to liquefaction and ever increasing cystic appearance within weeks. Neuroblastoma, whether solid or cystic, remains unchanged or might even increase in size. The fact that neuroblastoma tends to have such an excellent prognosis in the newborn offers an opportunity of waiting for a few weeks to watch for signs of change. MRI is excellent for the detection of hemorrhage, and at times a useful addition; and yet because of the possibility of a hemorrhagic neuroblastoma its contribution is less than that afforded by watching for possible changes by US, before committing the patient to further diagnostic procedures and treatment.

## Other neoplasms

Neoplasms of the neonatal adrenal glands other than neuroblastoma are extremely uncommon. Adrenocortical carcinoma has been described in the newborn, however[19]. Similarly pheochromocytoma occurs rarely in children and it is virtually non-existent in the neonatal period.

# References

1. Shackleford GD. Adrenal glands, pancreas and other retroperitoneal structures. In Siegel MJ, ed. *Pediatric Sonography*. New York: Raven Press, 1991:215
2. Oppenheimer DA, Caroll BA, Yousem S. Sonography of the normal neonatal adrenal gland. *Radiology* 1983;146:157–60
3. Bryan PJ, Caldamone AA, Morrison SC, *et al*. Ultrasound findings in the adreno-genital syndrome (congenital adrenal hyperplasia). *J Ultrasound Med* 1988;7:675–9
4. Grumbach MM, Conti FA. Disorders of sexual differentiation. In Wilson JD, Foster DS, eds. *Williams Textbook of Endocrinology*. Philadelphia: W.B. Saunders, 1985:315
5. Avni EF, Rypens F, Smet MH, *et al*. Sonographic demonstration of congenital adrenal hyperplasia in the neonate: the cerebriform pattern. *Pediatr Radiol* 1993;23:88–90
6. Sivit CJ, Hung W, Taylor GA, *et al*. Sonography in neonatal congenital adrenal hyperplasia. *Am J Radiol* 1991;156:141–3
7. Black J, Innes WD. Natural history of adrenal hemorrhage in the newborn. *Arch Dis Child* 1973;48:183–90
8. Currarino G, Wood B, Majd M. Diseases of the adrenal glands. In Silverman FN, Kuhn JP, eds. *Caffey's Pediatric X-ray Diagnosis: An Integrated Imaging Approach*, 9th edn, Vol. 2. St. Louis: Mosby, 1993, 1421
9. Atkinson GO, Kodroff MB, Gay BB, *et al*. Adrenal abscess in the neonate. *Radiology* 1985;155:101–4
10. McCauley RGK, Beckwith JB, Elias ER, *et al*. Benign hemorrhagic adrenocortical macrocyst in Beckwith–Wiedemann syndrome. *Am J Roentgen* 1991;157:549–52
11. Raafat F, Hashemian MP, Abrichami MA. Wolman's disease. Report of two new cases with a review of the literature. *Am J Clin Pathol* 1973;59:490–7
12. Kamolian N, Dudley AW, Beroukhim F. Wolman disease with jaundice and subarachnoid hemorrhage. *Am J Dis Child* 1973;126:671–5
13. Ellis JE, Patrick D. Wolman disease in a Pakistani infant. *Am J Dis Child* 1976;130:545–7
14. Lanzkowsky P. *Manual of Pediatric Hematology and Oncology*, 2nd edn. New York: Churchill Livingstone, 1995:419–36
15. Roshkow JE, Haller JO, Berdon WE, *et al*. Hirschsprung's disease, Ondine's curse and neuroblastoma-manifestations of neurocristopathy. *Pediatr Radiol* 1988;19:45–9
16. Forman HP, Leonidas JC, Berdon WE, *et al*. Congenital neuroblastoma: evaluation with multimodality imaging. *Radiology* 1990;175:365–8
17. Rosenfield NS, Leonidas JC, Barwick KW. Aggressive neuroblastoma simulating Wilms' tumor. *Radiology* 1988;166:165–7
18. Giulian BB, Chang CCN, Yoss BS. Prenatal ultrasonographic diagnosis of fetal adrenal neuroblastoma. *J Clin Ultrasound* 1986;14:225–7
19. Bulter H, Bick R, Morris MS. Unsuspected adrenal masses in the neonate: adrenal cortical carcinoma and neuroblastoma. *Pediatr Radiol* 1988;18:237–9.

## 7

# Abnormalities of the kidney: embryogenesis and radiologic appearance

*Joseph M. Silva, S. Zafar H. Jafri, Alexander A. Cacciarelli and Kathleen A. Barry*

## Embryology

Renal development progresses through three developmental stages: pronephros, mesonephros and metanephros. Human kidney formation originates within the cephalic portion of the intermediate mesoderm, which extends along the entire length of the dorsal body wall of the embryo[1]. During the late third to early fourth week of gestation, differentiation into pronephros (forekidney) occurs in the cervical region. Soon after, this non-functional collection of clustered cells and tubular-arranged structures degenerates and disappears[2].

During the fourth week of gestation, the involuting pronephros is replaced by the mesonephros (mid-kidney) (Figure 1). These develop immediately caudal to the pronephros and function as interim kidneys until the permanent kidneys are established[1,2]. The mesonephric uriniferous tubules arise from the laterally located, paired, nephrogenic cords. These tubules, which are associated with primitive functioning glomeruli, drain into the medially placed mesonephric (Wolffian) ducts which drain into the cloaca. Less than 40 mesonephric tubules are present in each kidney at any one time, and the mesonephros begins to regress near the end of the second month of gestation[2]. Remnants of the mesonephric duct persist in the male, serving as precursors of the vas deferens, seminal vesicles, and ejaculatory ducts. Remnants of the mesonephric tubules become the epididymis, parepididymis, and efferent ductules of the testes[3].

The metanephros (hind kidney), or permanent kidney, begins to develop during the fifth week of gestation (Figure 2). The permanent kidneys develop from two cell sources: the metanephric diverticulum (ureteral bud) and the metanephric blastema (nephrogenic mesoderm). The ureteral bud originates as a dorsal diverticulum from the mesonephric duct near its entry into the cloaca[4]. The ureteral bud grows toward and makes contact with the caudal end of the nephrogenic cord,

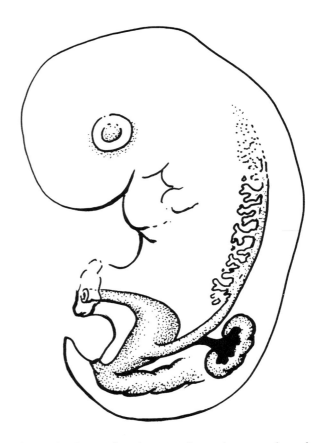

**Figure 1** Pronephros/mesonephros. At approximately the sixth fetal week, this shows the metanephric system developing as a bud off the mesonephric duct. The cloaca is present as a common communication between the developing urogenital and gastrointestinal systems

which becomes the metanephric blastema[5]. The ureteral bud is the primordium of the ureter, renal pelvis, calyces, and collecting tubules. Under the influence of the ureteral bud, the metanephric blastema is induced to develop into nephrons. Nephron formation will not occur in the absence of induction, whereas ureteral bud branching is dependent upon induction by the metanephric blastema. Following formation, the ureteral bud elongates and undergoes multiple divisions.

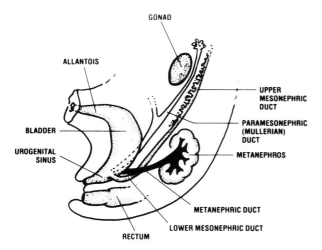

**Figure 2** Mesonephros/metanephros at approximately the seventh fetal week. Due to differential growth, the metanephric duct separates from the mesonephric duct and comes to enter the urogenital system more superiorly. The paramesonephric (müllerian) duct and mesonephric duct are developing but in an indifferent stage. Descent of a urorectal septum separates the urogenital and gastrointestinal tracts

Ureteral bud divisions are at first dichotomous, and the first four generations of tubules enlarge and become confluent, forming the renal pelvis; the second four generations coalesce to form the calyces. The remaining generations become the collecting tubules. The ends of the elongating collecting tubules induce clusters of metanephric blastema cells, which are of mesenchymal origin, to differentiate into metanephric vesicles. The metanephric vesicles elongate into S-shaped tubules that individually attach to collecting tubules at their proximal ends and form glomeruli at their distal ends. The distal free end of this tubule becomes the proximal end of the nephron; vascularization and invagination of the free end forms the glomerulus[1,2,4]. Further differentiation occurs with formation of functional units or nephron segments (the proximal and distal tubules).

Each nephron consists of a renal corpuscle (glomerulus and Bowman's capsule), proximal convoluted tubule, loop of Henle, and distal convoluted tubule (which contacts and becomes confluent with the collecting tubule). Ultrafiltration and urine production begin with vascularization of the glomerulus. By the third month of gestation, the nephrons formed are anatomically and histologically similar to those in the adult. As a result of the early branching of the ureteric bud and metanephric development, the

fetal kidney has a polylobar appearance (classically with 14 discrete renal lobes)[2,5].

The kidneys are initially located in the pelvis region, lying ventral to the sacrum. By nine weeks, they ascend and assume a more cranial adult position in the abdomen (Figure 3a,b). Initially, the

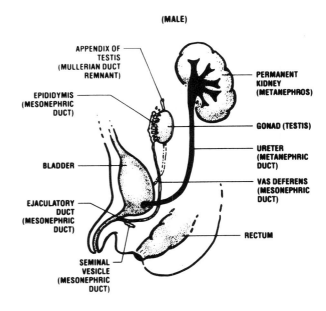

**Figure 3** (**a**) Metanephros (male) differentiation. The mesonephric duct forms the epididymis, vas deferens, ejaculatory duct, and seminal vesicles. The müllerian duct involutes and gives rise to the appendix of the testis and the prostatic uticle (not depicted)

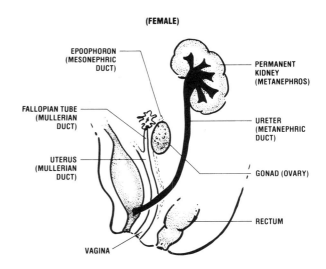

**Figure 3** (**b**) Metanephros (female) differentiation. The müllerian duct gives rise to the fallopian tubes, uterus, and upper vagina. The mesonephric duct involutes, giving rise to the epoophoron and Gartner's duct (not depicted)

renal hilum is ventral in position, but 90° medial rotation occurs with ascent so that the hilum is ultimately directed medially.

## Normal anatomy

Normal fetal kidneys should be routinely identified by 16 weeks menstrual age as paired hypoechoic, oval, paraspinal structures in the posterior mid-abdomen. Identification and sonographic appearance of the kidneys depend upon when the study is performed[6]. In the early to mid-second trimester, the hypoechoic renal cortex is poorly delineated from the renal sinus and perinephric tissues. By the middle to late second trimester, the kidneys are more readily visualized as echogenic perinephric fat accumulation delineates the renal outlines. At this stage, the central sinus region also becomes echogenic. By the mid-third trimester, the renal borders and central sinus become even more distinctly hyperechoic with identification of the hypoechoic pyramids and corticomedullary differentiation (Figure 4a,b). Various standards have been established for renal size as a function of menstrual age[7,8]. A commonly used rule of thumb is that renal length in millimeters approximates fetal menstrual age in weeks.

The fetal bladder should also be routinely identified by 16 weeks. Normally, the fetal bladder fills and empties every 30 to 45 minutes and bladder volume should change during the course of sonographic examination. The fetal bladder is thin-walled, and non-dilated fetal ureters are not routinely visualized.

Assessment of amniotic fluid volume is a critical step in evaluating renal function. Urine formation begins early in the second trimester. Prior to 16 weeks, the kidneys contribute little to amniotic fluid formation and thus a normal amount of fluid may be present in the absence of renal function. However, in the second half of pregnancy, fetal urine production is the source of most of the amniotic fluid[9].

Normal kidneys in newborns and young infants have several distinct sonographic features that differentiate them from the kidneys of older children and adults[10–12]. In neonates, the renal cortex is more echogenic, with echogenicity equal to liver and spleen. In pre-term infants, echogenicity may exceed that of the liver. Relatively increased cortical echogenicity is thought to result from glomeruli occupying a greater proportion of cortical volume, the greater proportional volume of the cellular component of the glomerular tuft,

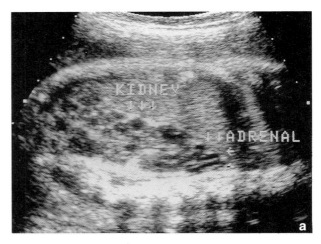

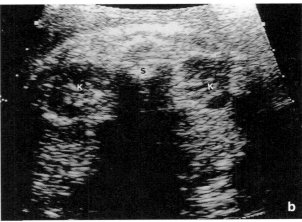

**Figure 4** (**a**) Sagittal scan at the level of the kidneys demonstrates normal fetal lobulation in the right kidney (K). Normal adrenal gland is also seen. (**b**) Axial scan at the level of the kidneys demonstrates normal renal cortex with echogenic renal sinus (K). S, Spine

and the location of 20% of the loops of Henle within the cortex as opposed to the medulla. In neonates and infants, the medullary pyramids are prominent, hypoechoic, and corticomedullary definition is accentuated resulting from a larger relative medullary volume. Lastly, echogenicity of the central sinus is reduced due to the paucity of renal sinus fat (Figure 5a,b). The renal cortex and medullary pyramids assume an adult pattern between one and six months of age and, by seven months, the renal parenchyma demonstrates an adult pattern[11]. The infant kidney contour is frequently lobulated resulting from residual fetal lobation. At the sites of fusion of embryonic renal lobes (renunculi) a parenchymal defect may be identified appearing as an echogenic triangular cortical defect in the anterosuperior or infero-posterior aspect of the kidney (junctional

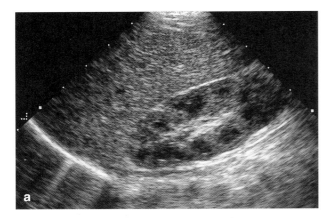

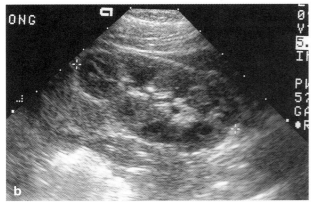

(**Figure 5** (**a**) Normal right renal ultrasound. (**b**) Normal left renal ultrasound

parenchymal defect) with an echogenic line extending from the defect to the renal sinus (intervenicular septum)[13,14]. This should not be confused with renal scar. Since normal renal length varies with age, several sonographic standards for renal length in infants and children have been established to aid in evaluation[15,16].

## Anomalies of number

### Renal agenesis

Congenital absence of renal tissue may result from failure of ureter bud development, early ureteric bud degeneration, failure of the bud to grow into and induce metanephric blastema, or via absence of metanephric blastema. In the case of failure of ureteral bud development, the ipsilateral trigone and ureteral orifice are absent (hemitrigone), whereas in the other instances a blind ending ureter of varying length may be present.

Bilateral renal agenesis (BRA) is rare, occurring in 1 to 2 per 10 000 births with a 2.5 : 1 male predominance[17]. The inheritance pattern and recurrence risk are complex with most cases being sporadic. BRA is incompatible with postnatal life, with neonatal death resulting from pulmonary hypoplasia secondary to oligohydramnios and uterine compression of the fetal thorax[18]. Infants exhibit characteristic features of Potter's syndrome including large low-set ears, prominent epicanthal folds, receding chin, flattened nose, and loose skin[19]. Sonographically, BRA is characterized by severe oligohydramnios, and non-visualization of the fetal bladder. The kidneys are not visualized; however, this may be difficult to confirm due to examination limitations secondary to severe oligohydramnios. The adrenal glands may enlarge and assume a reniform shape, or bowel in the renal fossa may mimic kidneys[20] (Figure 6). The renal arteries are also absent.

Unilateral renal agenesis is more common, occurring in 1 in 500 to 1 in 1500 births. This may be associated with congenital anomalies of the contralateral kidney and a variety of genital tract anomalies including unicornuate/bicornuate uterus, uterine and/or vaginal hypoplasia/aplasia in females, and seminal vesicle cysts, hypospadias, and vas deferens/testicular hypoplasia or aplasia in males[21,22] (Figure 7a,b). On sonography, a kidney is not identified within the renal fossa; however, renal ectopia must be excluded for a diagnosis of agenesis to be made. The renal artery and vein are absent or rudimentary. Ultrasound is also useful in delineating concomitant abnormalities involving the contralateral kidney and genital tract. If the contralateral kidney is functional, amniotic fluid volume and bladder filling will be normal. Again, care must be taken not to mistake an enlarged adrenal gland or bowel for kidney.

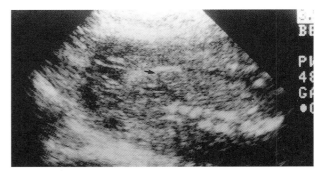

**Figure 6**  Reniform adrenal in renal agenesis. Longitudinal scan of the fetal abdomen shows the adrenal gland has conformed to the renal fossa (pseudo kidney) (arrows). In the absence of central sinus echoes and oligohydramnios, one should suspect renal agenesis. (Courtesy C. Comstock, MD, William Beaumont Hospital, Royal Oak, MI.)

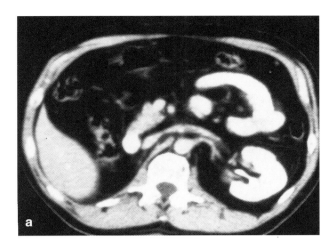

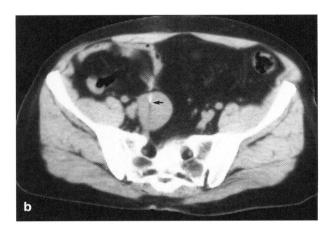

**Figure 7** Aplasia of the right kidney with ipsilateral seminal vesicle cyst. (**a**) CT scan at the level of the left renal artery and vein. There is absence of the right kidney and its associated vascular structures. (**b**) CT scan at the level of the mid sacrum. A well-defined, round, soft tissue density mass is seen. This was aspirated and the needle tip can be seen within the mass (arrow). This mass was found to represent a vesicle cyst

## Supernumerary kidney

Supernumerary kidney is an extra kidney distinct and separate from the normal kidney[23]. This extremely rare anomaly is seen with complete division or early branching of a ureteral bud. Most commonly, these kidneys are on the left, hypoplastic and positioned caudal to the normal kidneys[24] (Figure 8). A variety of associated genitourinary and non-genitourinary malformations have been reported.

## Anomalies of position, form, and orientation

### Pelvic kidney

Pelvic kidneys result from failure of ascent, usually with non-rotation. Blood supply is via adjacent vessels (e.g. iliac vessels/aorta). Bilateral pelvic kidneys may fuse to form a discoid or pancake kidney. In this condition, it is postulated that the two metanephroi are squeezed together between the umbilical arteries which may cause fusion and prevent ascent. Concomitant congenital anomalies have been reported including abnormal testicular descent, tetralogy of Fallot, vaginal agenesis, sacral agenesis, caudal regression, and anal anomalies[25]. Sonographic evaluation of the ectopic kidney may reveal abnormal shape, malrotation, or calyceal dilatation (Figure 9).

### Horseshoe kidney

Horseshoe kidney occurs in 1 in 500 to 1 in 1000 births and is two to three times more common in males. During migration, the two metanephroi come into contact with each other with subsequent partial fusion via either a parenchymal or, less commonly, fibrous isthmus which most commonly occurs in the lower poles. It has been suggested that this may result from mechanical pressure from the adjacent umbilical arteries, an abnormally placed umbilical artery, or abnormal migration of cells of the posterior intermediate mesoderm[5,26]. This isthmus is located between the aorta and inferior mesenteric artery, which prevents ascent and results in a characteristic lower lumbar location. There is associated bilateral malrotation with medially oriented lower poles and the pelvis and ureters being situated anterior to the renal parenchyma. Arterial supply arises from either the aorta or common iliac arteries. Increased incidence of hydronephrosis, calculi, and infection has been reported. While the likelihood of developing cancer in a horseshoe kidney does not differ from that in a normal kidney, the distribution of renal cancer differs markedly with Wilms' tumor and transitional cell carcinoma disproportionately represented[26–30]. Sonographic diagnosis is dependent upon identification of an isthmus of renal parenchyma crossing the midline, usually bridging medially oriented lower poles (Figure 10).

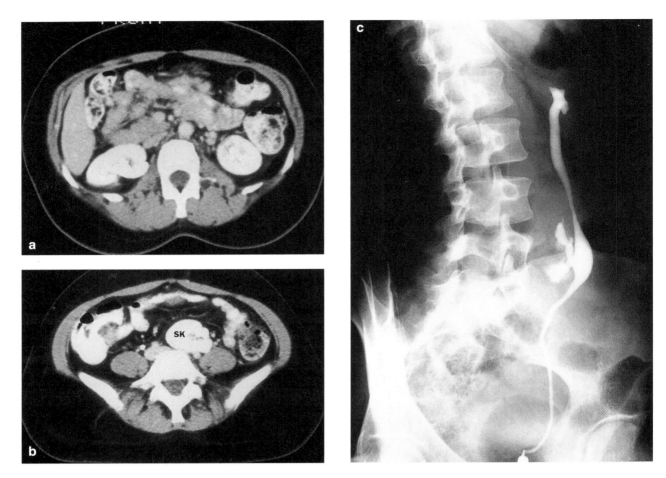

**Figure 8** Supernumerary kidney. (**a**) CT scan at the level of the kidneys. Both kidneys have a normal contour and orientation. (**b**) CT scan at the level of the iliac crests. Supernumerary kidney visualized at the level (SK). (**c**) Left retrograde pyelogram. The entire left ureter is filled with contrast. Two separate collecting systems can be seen, one in its normal location at the end of the ureter and the other at the level of the mid-ureter

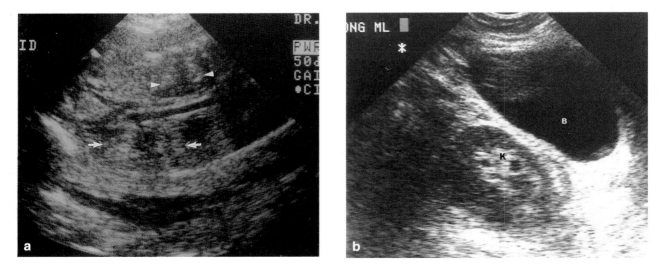

**Figure 9** Pelvic kidney. (**a**) Coronal scan of the fetal abdomen at the level of the iliac vessels demonstrates a left pelvic kidney (arrows). The right kidney is in normal location (arrowheads). (**b**) Sagittal sonogram of the pelvis demonstrates a left kidney (K) with parapelvic cysts. Urine filled bladder (B) is noted anteriorly. (Courtesy C. Comstock, MD, William Beaumont Hospital, Royal Oak, MI.)

## Crossed ectopy

Crossed ectopy occurs when a kidney is located on the opposite side of the midline from its ureteral orifice. This more commonly occurs in males and more commonly involves crossing of the left kidney to eventually lie on the right. The crossed kidney lies caudal to the normal kidney and may be fused or less commonly unfused to the normal kidney. The precise embryologic etiology is unknown. Theoretical explanations including faulty ureteral bud development with midline crossover to contact the contralateral metanephric blastema, vascular obstruction to renal ascent, and possibly teratogenic factors have been proposed[31]. While crossed ectopy is usually asymptomatic, patients may present with palpable mass or urinary tract symptoms. Associated urinary tract abnormalities include obstruction, calculus formation, infection, reflux, megaureter, hypospadias, urethral valves, and multicystic dysplasia. Non-urinary tract abnormalities include cryptorchidism, skeletal abnormalities, unilateral ovarian and fallopian tube agenesis, and a variety of gastrointestinal and cardiopulmonary anomalies[32]. Sonographically, both kidneys lie on the same side of the midline with no kidney in the contralateral renal fossa. With fusion, an enlarged reniform structure is identified with two renal sinuses. The fused lower pole unit is usually positioned medially, and a characteristic anterior and/or posterior notch may be seen at the fusion point[33] (Figure 11).

## Renal duplication

So-called renal duplication or 'duplex kidney' actually results from complete ureteral duplication. Its overall incidence ranges from 1.7 to 4.2%[34]. This occurs when a second ureteral bud arises from the mesonephric duct. The ureteral bud closest to the urogenital sinus drains the lower renal pole and enters the bladder at the trigone (orthotopic ureter), whereas the ureter draining the upper renal pole enters the bladder in a more medial and caudal position (ectopic ureter) and may be associated with a ureterocele. Less commonly, the upper pole ureter may insert outside the bladder especially in females. In these patients, the ureter may insert into the urethra, vagina, vestibule, or uterus in females and into the prostate urethra, seminal vesicles, vas deferens, epididymis, or ejaculatory duct in males. The orthotopic lower pole ureter is prone to vesicoureteral reflux due to its shortened ureteral tunnel at its bladder insertion at the trigone. This may result in scarring, atrophy, and decreased function of the lower pole. The ectopic upper pole ureter is prone to obstruction, with resultant hydronephrosis and decreased function of the upper pole.

Sonographically, complete separation of the central sinus echo complex into two discrete echodensities by normal parenchyma may be seen. With obstruction, asymmetric hydronephrosis will be present with dilatation of the upper pole moiety with parenchymal thinning and ureteral dilatation and preservation of a normal lower pole[35,36]. The

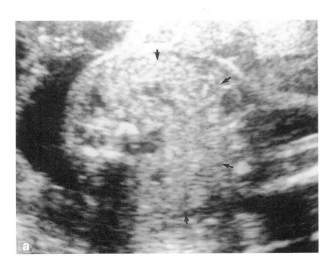

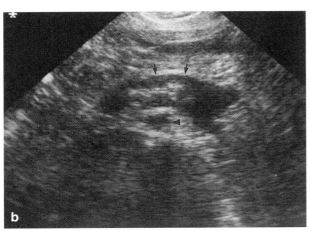

**Figure 10** Horseshoe kidney. (**a**) Axial scan of the fetal abdomen demonstrates large echogenic kidneys which appear contiguous across the midline in this trisomy 13 patient (arrows). (Courtesy Richard A. Bowerman, MD, Ann Arbor, MI.) (**b**) Transverse sonogram of the mid-abdomen demonstrates the hypoechoic isthmus of a horseshoe kidney (arrows). Abdominal aorta is noted posterior to the isthmus (arrowhead)

obstructed upper pole collecting system can mimic an upper pole cystic mass, while a dilated tortuous ectopic ureter may mimic a multi-septated cystic abdominal mass[37]. In any fetus or neonate suspected of having a duplicated collecting system, careful examination of the ureter and bladder must be performed for evaluation of associated ureteral dilatation and ectopic ureterocele (Figure 12). Ectopic ureteroceles present sonographically as anechoic, thin-walled masses of variable size and shape projecting into the lower bladder or urethra (Figure 13).

## Anomalies of differentiation

### Multicystic dysplastic kidney

Multicystic dysplastic kidney (MCDK) is a congenital, usually sporadic, renal dysplasia which is thought to be secondary to severe, generalized interference with ureteral bud function during early fetal life (before 8–10 weeks). It results from ureteral obstruction, and high ureteral atresia and pyelocaliceal occlusion are almost always present. *In utero*, obstruction interferes with ureteral bud

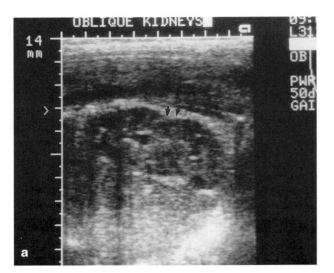

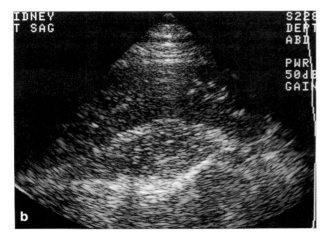

**Figure 11** Crossed fused ectopy. (a) Longitudinal oblique scan through the fetal abdomen demonstrates fused kidneys (arrows). (Courtesy B. Madrazo, MD, William Beaumont Hospital, Royal Oak, MI.) (b) Sagittal oblique sonogram of the right lower abdomen demonstrates ectopic left kidney fused with the lower pole of the right kidney. The left renal fossa was empty

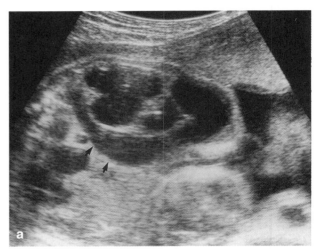

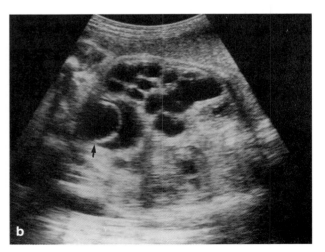

**Figure 12** Duplicated collecting system with ectopic ureterocele. (a) Coronal image of the abdomen demonstrates a duplex collecting system and dilated tortuous ureter (arrows). (b) In the same patient the sonogram demonstrates a very ectatic ureter and a large ureterocele as a cystic mass within the urinary bladder (arrow). (Courtesy of Richard A. Bowerman, MD, University of Michigan, Ann Arbor, MI.)

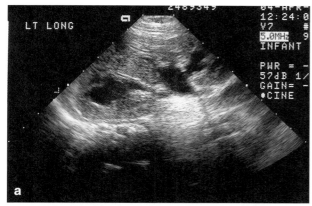

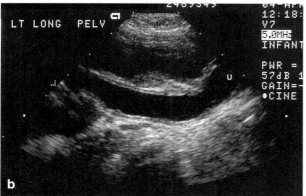

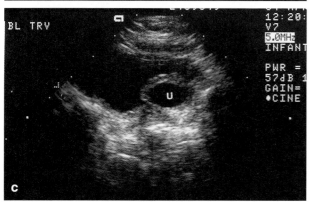

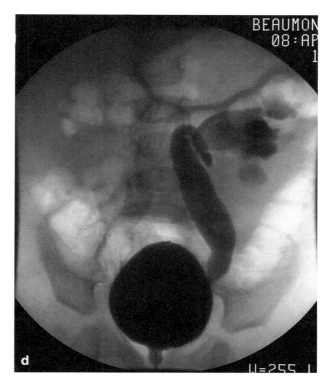

**Figure 13** (**a**) Sagittal sonogram in a neonate demonstrates a dilated duplicated collecting system of the left kidney. (**b**) Sagittal sonogram of the left side of the pelvis demonstrates an anechoic long tubular structure with a bulbous end consistent with a dilated ureter with ureterocele (U). (**c**) Transverse sonogram of the pelvis confirms a dilated left ureterocele (U) projecting into the urinary bladder. (**d**) Voiding cystourethrogram demonstrates a grade IV reflux into the lower pole collecting system of the same kidney

division and inhibits induction and maturation of nephrons[38,39]. The collecting tubules enlarge and become cystic, distorting the shape of the kidney, resulting in a collection of incompletely communicating, irregularly sized cysts with little or no functioning renal parenchyma. The ipsilateral renal artery is very small or absent. Contralateral abnormalities occur in approximately 40% of cases, most commonly ureteropelvic junction obstruction and vesicoureteral reflux. However, lethal anomalies such as bilateral MCDK and MCDK associated with contralateral agenesis are not uncommon[40,41]. MCDK is second only to hydronephrosis among causes of abdominal mass in the neonate.

Sonographic features include non-communicating cysts of varying sizes with non-medial location of the largest cyst, absence of identifiable renal pelvis or sinus, and absence of renal parenchyma surrounding the cysts[42] (Figure 14). Differentiation from severe hydronephrosis may be difficult both sonographically and scintigraphically (if hydronephrosis severely impairs renal function). Sonographic features helpful in the diagnosis of hydronephrosis include visible renal parenchyma surrounding a central cystic component, small peripheral cysts (calyces) budding off a large central cyst (pelvis), and visualization of a dilated ureter[43]. *In utero*, the MCDK may change markedly in size on serial examinations, with cyst enlargement and/or diminution presumably as a result of minimal residual glomerular filtration[44]. Amniotic fluid volume will depend upon the functional status of the contralateral kidney. A normal bladder filling and emptying suggests normal contralateral renal function, whereas oligohydramnios and diminished or absent bladder filling are seen with contralateral renal impairment, again stressing the importance of careful examination of the contralateral kidney in MCDK.

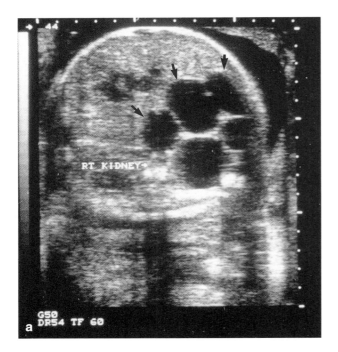

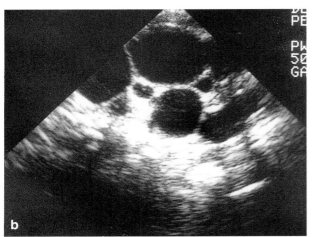

**Figure 14** Multicystic dysplastic kidney. (**a**) Transverse sonogram of the fetus upper abdomen demonstrates multiple round, fluid collections (arrows) consistent with multicystic dysplastic kidney. The contralateral normal kidney is noted. (Courtesy B. Madrazo, MD, William Beaumont Hospital, Royal Oak, MI.) (**b**) Sagittal sonogram of the left kidney demonstrates a large mass containing multiple round sonolucent areas and thick internal septations, consistent with multicystic dysplastic kidney. The contralateral kidney was normal

## Cystic renal dysplasia

Cystic renal dysplasia occurs most frequently in infants affected with urethral level obstruction during nephrogenesis. It may also occur secondary to uretero-pelvic junction or uretero-vesicle junction obstruction. The type and severity of dysplasia depends on the time in fetal life that the obstruction develops. The multicystic dysplastic kidney results from an early developmental obstruction, whereas cystic renal dysplasia results from an obstructive phenomenon developing later in fetal life as a result of posterior urethral valves. The prenatal sonographic findings of cystic renal dysplasia demonstrate renal cortical cysts in the setting of obstructive uropathy. Dysplastic kidneys also tend to have increased echogenicity (Figure 15).

## Recessive polycystic kidney disease

Recessive polycystic kidney disease (RPCKD) is relatively uncommon, occurring in 1 in 6000 to 14 000 births with a 2 : 1 female predominance, and is transmitted by autosomal recessive inheritance[45]. It is characterized by diffuse enlargement, sacculations, and cystic diverticula of the collecting tubules. Embryologically, the ureteral bud and metanephric blastema are normal and normal nephron formation occurs. However, during the later half of intrauterine life, the

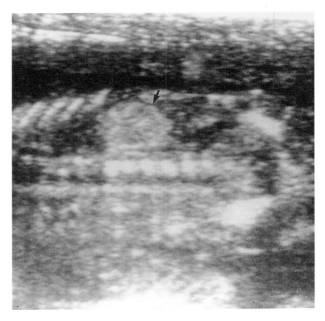

**Figure 15** Coronal scan through the fetal abdomen demonstrates a very echogenic kidney secondary to multiple tiny cortical cysts (arrow). (Courtesy C. Comstock, MD, William Beaumont Hospital, Royal Oak, MI.)

collecting tubules of both kidneys undergo dilatation with irregular formation of saccules and diverticula[46]. The exact pathogenesis is not known. These dilated tubules are not visualized sonographically, but the numerous tubular wall – fluid interfaces produce renal hyperechogenicity. Thus, the sonographic findings include bilateral renal enlargement, diffuse increased echogenicity, and loss of definition of the renal sinus, medulla and cortex[47,48]. *In utero*, diagnosis relies on the demonstration of bilaterally enlarged echogenic kidneys often with oligohydramnios. The diagnosis may be made at 16–18 weeks, especially if oligohydramnios or non-visualization of the bladder are present. However, the *in utero* appearance varies depending on severity of involvement and the aforementioned findings may not become apparent until the third trimester (Figure 16).

RPCKD is associated with biliary ectasia and hepatic fibrosis, the severity of which is usually inversely proportional to the degree of renal involvement[49] (Figure 17). In infants, renal disease predominates with renal failure and minimal or no hepatic findings. In older children, hepatic findings predominate with hepatic fibrosis and portal hypertension which may manifest sonographically as diffusely increased hepatic echogenicity and biliary ductal ectasia.

## Dominant polycystic kidney disease

Dominant polycystic kidney disease (DPCKD) is transmitted by autosomal dominant inheritance and usually presents secondary to pain, hypertension, or hematuria in the fourth decade[50]. Incidence based on autopsy studies ranges from 1 per 350 to 1 per 620[45]. While perinatal presentation is rare, DPCKD may occur in the neonate.

Cyst formation is secondary to hyperplasia of tubular and ductal epithelial cells, perhaps with secondary obstruction, giving rise to cysts that may occur in any part of the nephron or collecting tubule[51]. Cysts of varying sizes are present throughout the cortex and medulla interspersed with normal parenchyma. DPCKD is associated with cysts in multiple organs, most commonly liver and pancreas, but also spleen, ovaries, testes, epididymis, seminal vesicles, thyroid, lung, uterus and bladder, as well as saccular aneurysms of the cerebral arteries. There is an increased incidence of renal cell carcinoma in patients with DPCKD[52]. Sonographically, the fetus or neonate demonstrates enlarged, homogeneously echogenic kidneys

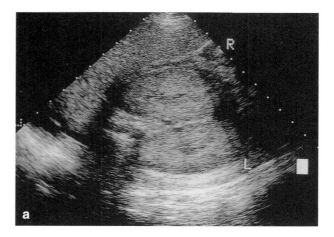

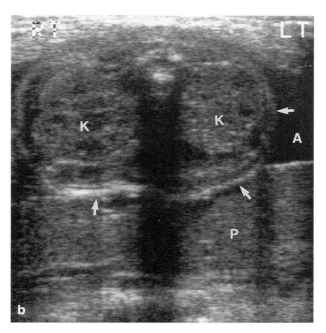

**Figure 16** Autosomal recessive polycystic kidney disease. (**a**) Coronal oblique scan of a fetus with bilateral echogenic enlarged kidneys which meet in the midline. The hyperechoic texture is due to the multiple interfaces generated by the walls of the microscopic cysts. (Courtesy C. Comstock, MD, William Beaumont Hospital, Royal Oak, MI.) (**b**) Transverse sonogram of the fetal abdomen reveals large echogenic kidneys (K) which occupy most of the abdominal cavity (arrows). There is associated oligohydramniosis. A, amniotic fluid; P, placenta; K, kidney. (Courtesy B. Madrazo, MD, William Beaumont Hospital, Royal Oak, MI.)

with loss of corticomedullary differentiation (Figure 18). Hyperechogenicity results from interfaces of multiple tiny cysts in addition, small discrete cysts may be seen.

Sonographic findings are similar to RPCKD; however, lack of significant renal impairment,

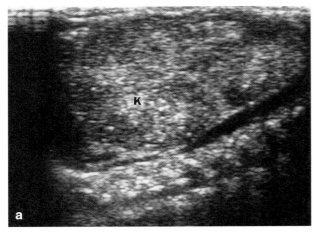

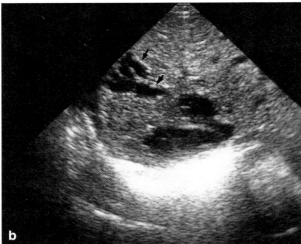

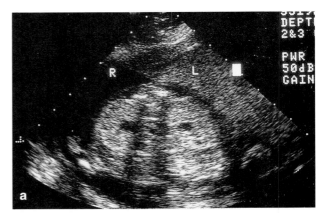

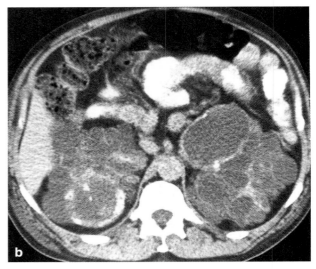

**Figure 17** Recessive polycystic kidney with biliary ectasia. (a) Sagittal sonogram of the left kidney in a newborn reveals an enlarged kidney (measuring 9.8 cm in length) (K). The kidney is echogenic with obliteration of the normal corticomedullary and central sinus differentiation. (b) Subxyphoid transverse sonogram in the same child reveals biliary ductal ectasia in the right lobe of the liver (arrows)

**Figure 18** Dominant polycystic kidney disease. (a) Fetal sonogram demonstrates enlarged echogenic kidneys with multiple small sonolucencies consistent with small cysts. (Courtesy C. Comstock, MD, William Beaumont Hospital Royal Oak, MI). (b) Abdominal CT in the grandfather of the above fetus demonstrates an appearance typical of dominant polycystic kidney disease. Patient underwent bilateral nephrectomy

normal amniotic fluid volume, family history, or histologic sampling allows differentiation. In older children, renal enlargement with multiple discrete cysts are identified as in adults.

## Glomerulocystic disease

Glomerulocystic disease (GCD) is a rare congenital renal abnormality which is usually sporadic and is characterized histologically by uniform cystic dilatation of Bowman's spaces in the renal cortex. In this form of cystic disease, clinical presentation and prognosis are extremely variable[53]. There may be associated small peripheral hepatic cysts and

adenomas. Sonographically, GCD is similar to RPCKD and neonatal DPCKD with enlarged echogenic kidneys, loss of corticomedullary differentiation, and occasionally small (<1 cm) cortical cysts are seen[54,55] (Figure 19).

## Medullary cystic disease

Medullary cystic disease is usually diagnosed clinically based on findings of polyuria, polydipsia, renal salt wasting, hyposthenuria, anemia, and progressive azotemia. Clinical onset occurs after 3 to 5 years of age and most commonly is in adolescence. It has been classified into two types by

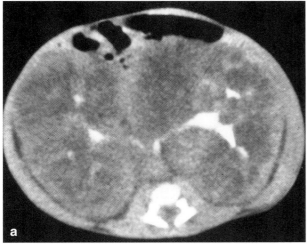

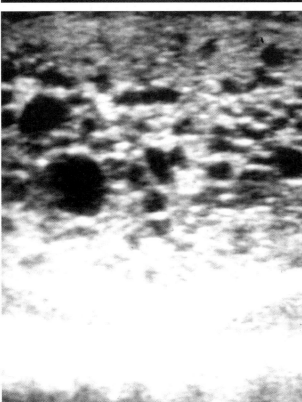

**Figure 19** Glomerulocystic disease. (a) Computed tomography obtained following intravenous contrast injection in a newborn demonstrates bilateral multiple renal cysts and compressed renal collecting system. (b) Longitudinal sonogram in the first week of life demonstrates markedly enlarged kidneys with multiple anechoic cysts of varying size. The normal cortico-medullary distinction was not present, and renal pyramids could not be identified. Renal biopsy established the diagnosis of glomerulocystic kidney disease. (Courtesy J.P. Kuhn, MD, Children's Hospital, Buffalo, NY.)

age at onset. The adult onset type is transmitted in an autosomal dominant fashion, presenting in young adults with rapidly progressive renal failure. The juvenile onset type (juvenile nephronophthisis) is transmitted by autosomal recessive inheritance and is characterized by more slowly progressive renal failure.

Pathologic features include normal sized to slightly small kidneys with cortical thinning, small medullary and corticomedullary junction cysts arising from the loops of Henle and collecting tubules, interstitial fibrosis, periglomerular fibrosis, and tubular atrophy[56,57]. Sonographic findings include the presence of a few small (< 2 cm) medullary or corticomedullary cysts in normal sized or moderately small kidneys, loss of corticomedullary differentiation, and increased parenchymal echogenicity[57,58].

*Renal cystic disease associated with hereditary syndromes*

A variety of hereditary syndromes are associated with renal cysts. These include Meckel–Gruber syndrome (occipital encephalocele, microcephaly, polydactyly), Zellweger syndrome (cerebrohepato-renal syndrome), Jeune's asphyxiating thoracic dystrophy, Conradi syndrome (chondrodysplasia punctata), oro-facial-digital syndrome, Turner's syndrome, tuberous sclerosis, and von Hippel–Lindau syndrome.

Tuberous sclerosis (Bourneville's disease) is autosomal dominant with a relatively high rate of new mutations. It is characterized by mental retardation, seizures and hamartomas of multiple organs. Renal cystic disease (multiple cortical and medullary simple cysts) is a common manifestation. Hamartomas may be seen in the central nervous system (CNS) (periventricular and cortical tubers), skin (adenoma sebaceum), retina (phakoma), heart (rhabdomyoma), bone (bone island), and kidney (angiomyolipoma). Up to 80% of patients have renal angiomyolipomas which are usually multiple and bilateral[59] (Figure 20).

Von Hippel–Lindau syndrome (VHL) is also transmitted by an autosomal dominant gene. Multiple bilateral cortical renal cysts, usually presenting in adulthood, are seen in approximately 75% of cases. Renal cell carcinoma, which may be multicentric or bilateral occurs in 30–40%[60]. VHL is also associated with CNS and retinal hemangioblastomas, pheochromocytomas and cysts and tumors of other organs (including pancreas, liver and epididymis)[61] (Figure 21).

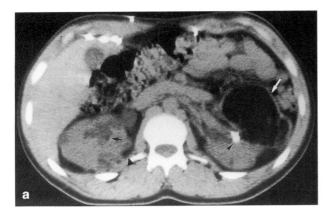

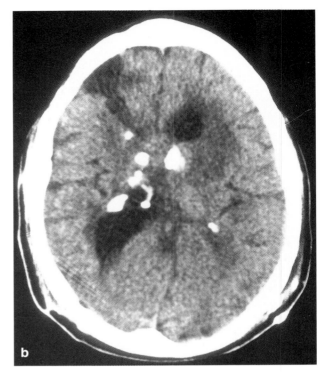

**Figure 20** Tuberous sclerosis. (**a**) Unenhanced CT at the level of the kidneys demonstrates a large, predominantly fatty mass within the left kidney, consistent with angiomyolipoma (arrow). Incidental renal calculus is also present (arrowhead). Numerous right renal cysts (arrow) are also seen, as well as a second smaller angiomyolipoma (arrowhead). (**b**) Unenhanced HCT demonstrates multiple calcified subependymal nodules, consistent with multiple calcified hamartomas (tubers)

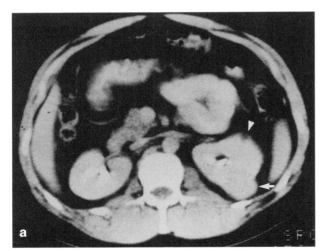

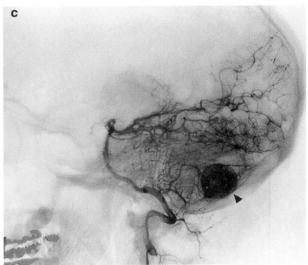

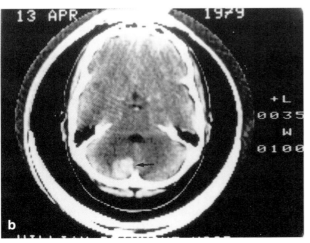

**Figure 21** Von Hippel – Landau disease. (**a**) Enhanced CT scan at the level of the kidneys demonstrates a solid mass within the left kidney (arrow), representing surgically proven renal cell carcinoma. A small simple cyst is also seen (arrowhead). (**b**) Contrast-enhanced HCT in the same patient demonstrates an enhancing cerebellar mass (arrow). (**c**) This was hypervascular on angiography (arrowhead) and was a proven cerebellar hemangioblastoma. (With permission, D.P. Wesolowski, *et al.*[61])

# References

1. Carlson BM. The development of the urogenital system. In *Patterns Foundation of Embryology*. New York: McGraw-Hill, 1981:440–76

2. Pansky B. The urinary system. In *Review of Medical Embryology*, Unit 8. New York: MacMillan, 1982: 246–83

3. Davidson AJ, Hartman DS. Radiologic anatomy of the kidney and ureter. In *Radiology of the Kidney and Urinary Tract*, 2nd edn. Philadelphia: W.B. Saunders, 1994:53–64

4. Moore KL. The urogenital system. In *The Developing Human*, 4th edn. Philadelphia: W.B. Saunders Company, 1988:246–83

5. Dunnick NR, McCallum RW, Sandler CM. Anatomy and embryology. In *Textbook of Uroradiology*. Baltimore: Williams and Wilkins, 1991:10–13

6. Bowie JD, Rosenberg ER, Andreotti RF, *et al*. The changing sonographic appearance of fetal kidneys during pregnancy. *J Ultrasound Med* 1983;2:505–7

7. Jeanty P, Dramaix-Wilmet M, Elkhazen N. Measurement of fetal kidney growth on ultrasound. *Radiology* 1982;144:159–62

8. Sagi J, Vagman I, David MP, *et al*. Fetal kidney size related to gestational age. *Gynecol Obstet Invest* 1987; 23:1–4

9. Seeds AE. Current concepts of amniotic fluid dynamics. *Am J Obstet Gynecol* 1980;138:575–86

10. Hricak H, Slovis T, Callen C, *et al*. Neonatal kidneys: sonographic anatomic correlation. *Radiology* 1983; 147:699–702

11. Han B, Babcock D. Sonographic measurements and appearance of normal kidneys in children. *Am J Radiol* 1995;145:611–16

12. Haller J, Berdon W, Friedman A. Increased renal cortical echogenicity: a normal finding in neonates and infants. *Radiology* 1982;142:173–4

13. Kenney I, Wild S. The renal parenchymal junctional line in children: ultrasonic frequency and appearances. *Br J Radiol* 1987;60:865–8

14. Carter A, Horgan J, Jennings T, *et al*. The junctional parenchymal defect: a sonographic variant of renal anatomy. *Radiology* 1985;154:499–502

15. Blane C, Bookstein F, DiPietro M, *et al*. Sonographic standards for normal infant kidney length. *Am J Radiol* 1985;145:1289–91

16. Rosenbaum D, Korngold E, Teele R. Sonographic assessment of renal length in normal children. *Am J Radiol* 1984;142:467–69

17. Sangel P, Feinstein S, Chandra P, *et al*. Recurrent bilateral renal agenesis. *Am J Obstet Gynecol* 1986;155:1078–79

18. Marres A, Mereu G, Dessi C, *et al*. Oligohydramnios and extrarenal abnormalities in Potter syndrome. *J Pediatr* 1983;102:597–8

19. Potter E. Bilateral absence of ureters and kidneys. A report of 50 cases. *Obstet Gynecol* 1965;25:3–12

20. McGahan JP, Myracle MR. Adrenal hypertrophy: possible pitfall in the sonographic diagnosis of renal agenesis. *J Ultrasound Med* 1986;5:265–8

21. Sayer T, O'Reilly P. Bicornuate and unicornuate uterus associated with unilateral renal aplasia and abnormal solitary kidneys: report of three cases. *J Urol* 1986;135:110–11

22. Heaney JA, Pfister RC, Mecres EM. Giant cyst of the seminal vesicle with renal agenesis. *Am J Radiol* 1987;149:139–40

23. Peterson R. Kidney. In *Urologic Pathology*. Philadelphia: J.B. Lippincott, 1992:1–30

24. N'Guessan G, Stephens F. Supernumerary kidney. *J Urol* 1983;130:649–53

25. Goren E, Eidelman A. Pelvic cake kidney drained by a single ureter. *Urology* 1987;30:492–3

26. Blackard C, Mellinger T. Cancer in a horseshoe kidney. *Arch Surg* 1968;97:616–27

27. Nirgiotis J, Black C, Sherman J. Wilm's tumor in horseshoe kidney: presentation due to ureteropelvic junction obstruction. *J Surg Oncol* 1991;48:210–12

28. Smith-Behn J, Memo R. Malignancy in horseshoe kidney. *South Med J* 1988;81:1451–52

29. Buntley D. Malignancy associated with horseshoe kidney. *Urology* 1976;8:146–8

30. Hohenfellner M, Schultz-Lampel D, Lampel A, *et al*. Tumor in the horseshoe kidney. Clinical implications and review of embryogenesis. *J Urol* 1992;147:1098–1102

31. Hertz M, Rubinstein Z, Shahin N, *et al*. Crossed renal ectopia: clinical and radiological findings in 22 cases. *Clin Radiol* 1977;28:339–44

32. Felzenberg J, Nasrallah P. Crossed renal ectopia without fusion associated with hydronephrosis in an infant. *Urology* 1991;38:450–2

33. McCarthy S, Rosenfield A. Ultrasonography in crossed renal ectopia. *J Ultrasound Med* 1984;3: 107–12

34. Schaffer R, Shih Y, Becker J. Sonographic identification of collecting system duplications. *J Clin Ultrasound* 1983;11:309–12

35. Jeffrey RB, Laing F, Wing V, *et al*. Sonography of the fetal duplex kidney. *Radiology* 1984;153:123–4

36. Mascatello V, Smith E, Larrera G, *et al*. Ultrasonic evaluation of the obstructed duplex kidney. *Am J Roentgenol* 1977;129:113–20

37. Nussbaum A, Dorst J, Jeffs R, *et al*. Ectopic ureter and ureterocele: their varied sonographic manifestations. *Radiology* 1986;159:227–35

38. Potter EL. Type II cystic kidney: early ampullary inhibition. In *Normal and Abnormal Development of the Kidney*. Chicago: Yearbook Medical Publishers, 1972;154–81

39. Beck D. The effect of intrauterine urinary obstruction upon the development of the fetal kidney. *J Urol* 1971;105:784–9

40. Atiyeh B, Husmann D, Baum M. Contralateral renal abnormalities in multicystic dysplastic kidney disease. *J Pediatr* 1992;121:65–7

41. Kleiner B, Filly R, Mack L, *et al*. Multicystic dysplastic kidney: observation of contralateral disease on the fetal population. *Radiology* 1986;161:27–9

42. Stuck K, Kuff S, Silver T. Ultrasonic features of multicystic dysplastic kidney: expanded diagnostic criteria. *Radiology* 1982;143:217–21

43. Sanders R, Hartman D. The sonographic distinction between neonatal multicystic kidney and hydronephrosis. *Radiology* 1984;151:621–5

44. Hashimoto B, Filly R, Taylor P. Multicystic dysplastic kidney *in utero*: changing appearance on ultrasound. *Radiology* 1986;159:107–9

45. Bosniak M, Ambos M. Polycystic kidney disease. *Sem Roentgenol* 1975;10:133–43

46. Cole BR. Autosomal recessive polycystic kidney disease. In Gardner KD, Bernstein J, eds. *The Cystic Kidney*. Boston: Kluwer Academic Publishers, 1990: 327–50

47. Boal D, Teele R. Sonography of infantile polycystic kidney disease. *Am J Radiol* 1980;135:575–80

48. Kaariainen H, Jaaskelsinen J, Kiuisaari L. Dominant and recessive polycystic kidney disease in children: classification by intravenous pyelography, ultrasound, and computed tomography. *Pediatr Radiol* 1988;18:45–50

49. Six R, Oliphant M, Grossman H. A spectrum of renal tubular ectasia and hepatic fibrosis. *Radiology* 1975;117:117–22

50. Gabow P, Schrier R. Pathophysiology of adult polycystic kidney disease. *Adv Nephrol* 1989;18:19–32

51. Gabow P. Autosomal dominant polycystic kidney disease. In Gardner KD Jr, Bernstein J, eds. *The Cystic Kidney*. Boston: Kluwer Academic Publishers, 1990:295–26

52. Goldman SM, Hartman D. Autosomal dominant polycystic kidney disease. In Hartman DS, ed. *Renal Cystic Disease, AFIP Atlas of Radiologic Pathologic Correlation. Fascicle 1*. Philadelphia: W.B. Saunders Co., 1989:88–107

53. Cachero S, Montgomery P, Seidel F, *et al*. Glomerulocystic kidney disease: case report. *Pediatr Radiol* 1990;20:491–3

54. Fredericks B, de Camp M, Chow C, *et al*. Glomerulocystic renal disease: ultrasound appearances. *Pediatr Radiol* 1989;19:184–6

55. Fitch S, Stapleton F. Ultrasonographic features of glomerulocystic disease in infancy: similarity to infantile polycystic kidney disease. *Pediatr Radiol* 1986;16:400–2

56. Lang E. Roentgenologic assessment of medullary cysts. *Sem Roentgenol* 1975;10:145–54

57. Wood B. Renal cystic disease in infants and children. *Urol Radiol* 1992;14:284–95

58. Garel L, Habib R, Pariente D, *et al*. Juvenile nephronophthisis: sonographic appearance in children with severe uremia. *Radiology* 1984;151:93–6

59. Mitnick J, Bosniak M, Hilton S, *et al*. Cystic renal disease in tuberous sclerosis. *Radiology* 1983;147:85–7

60. Hartman D. Renal cystic disease in multisystemic conditions. *Urol Radiol* 1992;14:13–17

61. Wesolowski D, Ellwood R, Schwab K, *et al*. Von Hippel–Lindau syndrome in identical twins: case reports. *Br J Radiol* 1981;54:982–6

# Neonatal hydronephrosis

## 8

*Carrie Ruzal-Shapiro*

The evaluation of the young infant's kidneys requires an appreciation of the differences between the adult kidney and that of the infant and young child (Figure 1). The cortex of the young child's kidney is hyperechoic relative to that of the adult, and is close in echotexture to that of the spleen or liver, rather than being hypoechoic compared to them as in the adult. In addition, the pyramids are relatively prominent and hypoechoic. There is also a paucity of renal sinus fat resulting in a less echogenic renal sinus. The prominent pyramids should not be mistaken for dilated calyces and hydronephrosis (Figure 2)[1–5].

Hydronephrosis means dilatation of the collecting system. Although hydronephrosis most commonly is due to obstruction, there are other causes of dilatation of the collecting system. These include reflux and the ectasia of prune belly syndrome, as well as a variety of other conditions. Hydronephrosis is identified by observing anechoic cystic structures (calyces) which connect to a central dilated cyst (the renal pelvis) (Figure 3)[6–11]. This must be distinguished from the non-communicating cysts of multi-cystic dysplastic kidneys (Figures 4 and 5a,b)[12]. When performing ultrasound examinations, it is important to look for

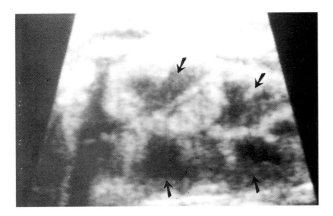

**Figure 1** Normal right kidney longitudinal view in a 1-day-old, arrows point to hypoechoic pyramids

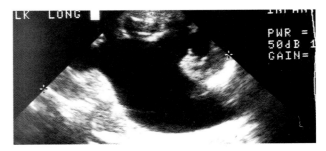

**Figure 3** Hydronephrosis secondary to ureteropelvic junction obstruction; longitudinal image showing communication of anechoic dilated calyces with pelvis

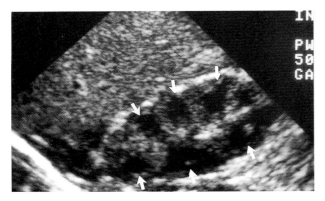

**Figure 2** Arrows point to extremely large hypoechoic pyramids in normal infant (longitudinal view)

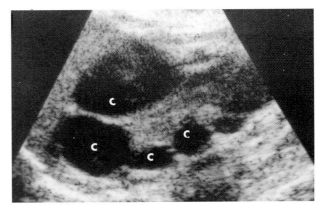

**Figure 4** Multicystic dysplastic kidney; longitudinal images showing multiple non-connecting anechoic cysts (c)

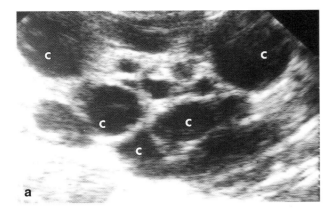

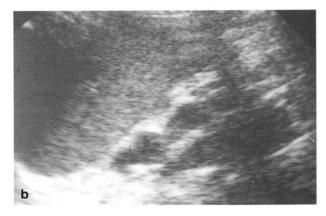

**Figure 5** (**a**) Multicystic kidney, day 1 of life; longitudinal image showing multiple non-connecting cysts (C). (**b**) Multicystic dysplastic kidney showing resorption of fluid with residual small cysts and dysplastic tissue at 13 months of age

a dilated ureter. This helps to distinguish obstruction at the level of the ureteropelvic junction from other causes of hydronephrosis such as ureterovesical obstruction and reflux[8,13,14].

## Ureteropelvic junction obstruction

Ureteropelvic junction (UPJ) obstruction is the most common cause of hydronephrosis in the neonate. The etiology is controversial, but it is generally believed to be due most commonly to an intrinsic stenosis which is congenital in nature. In some cases, there is no mechanical obstruction but a hypoplasia of local ureteral musculature resulting in a failure of peristalsis and a functional obstruction. Ureteral kinks and high insertion of the ureter are often found but are generally

believed to be secondary findings. The disease is generally unilateral, with only about 10% of patients having contralateral UPJ obstruction at presentation. Some patients appear to have a narrow but non-obstructed contralateral pelvic junction. These children may progress to a more apparent UPJ obstruction over time[13-16].

Before the advent of routine prenatal screening, UPJ obstruction was generally diagnosed after the pediatrician palpated an abdominal mass in a neonate. Older children presented with hematuria, flank pain after fluid challenge, urinary tract infections, and occasionally sepsis. Currently many cases are identified incidentally on prenatal ultrasound.

Ultrasound is used to diagnose the presence of pylocaliectasis. A central anechoic structure representing the pelvis is seen connecting to surrounding cystic areas representing dilated calyces. The central cyst may extend outside of the kidney. The normal ureter is generally not appreciated. The degree of distention should be evaluated as well as the appearance of the echotexture of the kidneys. This varies from a normal appearance without noticeable scarring to a thin, barely perceptible shell of parenchyma. The parenchyma may be markedly echogenic and contain cortical cysts representing a dysplasia due to obstruction. Evaluation of the pelvis using a full bladder as a sonic window is performed to exclude ureteral dilatation which should suggest more distal obstruction or reflux as the cause of the hydronephrosis. Morphology can be well described using ultrasound, but additional techniques such as intravenous urography or nuclear scanning are needed to evaluate function and the degree of obstruction[17-26].

There is a lack of consensus on the evaluation of babies with the diagnosis of prenatal hydronephrosis. It is clear that all babies with significant prenatal hydronephrosis should have postnatal scans, but the definition of significant hydronephrosis is not agreed upon by obstetrical sonographers, and the optimum timing of follow-up scans is still unclear. Early after birth, significant hydronephrosis from UPJ obstruction can be missed due to the relative oliguria of the first few days of life. At our institution, if the prenatal ultrasound demonstrates moderately severe unilateral or bilateral hydronephrosis, we scan the patient prior to discharge from the nursery (at day 1 or 2 of life). If abnormalities are detected, appropriate work-up such as nuclear scanning or voiding cystourethrography is performed. Babies who have obstruction can be sent home from the hospital on prophylactic antibiotics to avoid stasis-induced infection while waiting for definitive therapy[23,24]. If the scan appears normal, the patient returns at three months, six months and one year of age for follow-up ultrasound examinations (Figure 6a,b)[25]. If the scan remains normal, one additional scan at five to six years of age is advised. If the prenatal scan shows mild hydronephrosis, the first follow-up ultrasound is done at two weeks of age. If this is normal, the imaging either stops or one additional exam is done between three and six months of age.

## Megaureter

Megaureters are dilated, tortuous ureters that may be seen in various conditions. We add descriptive names to help divide and classify the different types of megaureter. They may be idiopathic or due to obstruction or reflux. They are further classified as primary or secondary. Primary obstructive megaureter occurs at the uretero-vesicle junction or just above it[27,28]. In the latter instance, it is a functional obstruction due to the inability of this portion of ureter to transmit a peristaltic wave. In secondary obstructing mega-ureter, the ureteral dilatation may be due to a neurogenic bladder or bladder outlet obstruction such as is seen in the presence of posterior urethral valves. Ectopically inserted ureters with or without ureteroceles may result in marked ureterectasia[29].

Refluxing megaureter is due to an abnormality in the tunneling of the distal ureter through the bladder wall. Secondary or exacerbating causes of reflux include neurogenic bladder and posterior urethral valves. The presence of reflux is difficult to determine using standard ultrasound techniques. Static ultrasound images often underestimate the degree of reflux: if reflux is mild the ultrasound may look perfectly normal (Figure 7)[30–32].

Primary non-obstructive, non-refluxing mega-ureter is idiopathic and a diagnosis of exclusion. It may involve a portion or the entire ureter.

## Duplication of the renal collecting system

Ureteral duplication is the most common anomaly of the genitourinary system. Approximately 1 in 125 patients are affected. The right and left kidneys are affected with equal frequency. Approximately 40% of patients have bilateral

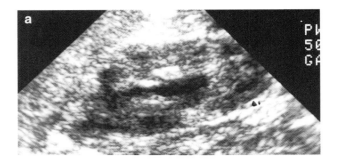

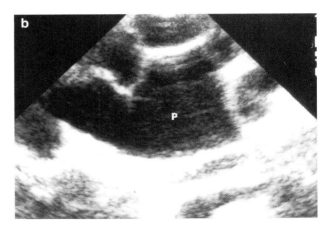

**Figure 6** (a) Initial longitudinal image in newborn with moderate prenatal hydronephrosis (day 1 of life) shows minimal dilatation of collecting system and no evidence of parenchymal thinning. (b) At three months of age the follow-up longitudinal US in this same baby shows marked dilatation of the collecting system and thinning of the parenchyma (ureteropelvic junction obstruction), (P, dilated pelvis)

duplications. The duplications often are asymmetric. Duplication represents a spectrum of changes. A bifid pelvis may be thought of as representing the most minimal form of duplication, while in complete duplication the ureters enter the bladder separately. The ureters may join together anywhere along their course. Occasionally the two ureters join within the bladder wall and have a common opening. The portion of the kidney drained by the lower pole system usually is larger than the upper pole segment[33,34].

When the kidney is completely duplicated, two separate pelvocalyceal systems drain into two separate ureters, each having its own insertion into the bladder. The two openings generally are in one common sheath. The relationship of the insertion sites of the distal ureters is constant. The ureter from the upper pole moiety typically enters the bladder more caudally and more medially than the ureter draining the lower pole segment. This is

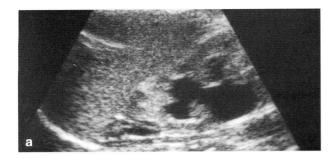

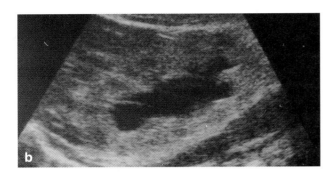

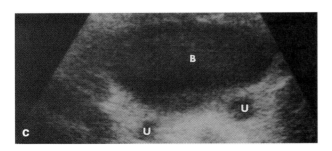

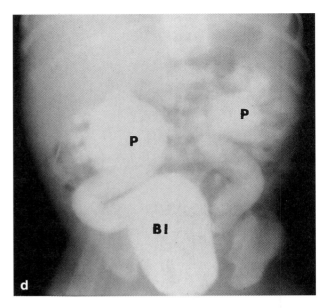

**Figure 7 (a – d)** Longitudinal views of both kidneys show mild – moderate hydronephrosis. Transverse image of the bladder reveals ureteral dilatation bilaterally suggesting megaureter. Voiding cystourethrogram reveals high grade reflux. Note how USG underestimates degree of reflux. (B, bladder; U, ureter; Bl, bladder; P, renal pelvis)

known as the Weigert-Meyer Rule. Ureteral ectopia is a common consequence of duplications. In either sex, the upper pole ureter may enter the bladder inferomedially to the trigone or the bladder neck. In girls, it may also end ectopically in the vestibule, vagina, or urethra. In boys, the ectopic termination may be in the posterior urethra or seminal vesicles. In girls, the ureter may end distal to the external sphincter, and the patient presents with dribbling. Patients with obstruction present with signs of infection. The upper pole ureter commonly ends in a uretero-cele, resulting in various degrees of obstruction. Congenital ureteropelvic junction obstructions may occur in the setting of renal duplications. They are most likely to involve the lower pole. Reflux is a common occurrence, predominantly but not exclusively involving the lower pole moiety due to the distortion of tunneling through the bladder wall. Reflux may result in scarring in the lower pole segment. Obstruction of the upper pole

may result in severe thinning of the upper pole parenchyma. A markedly dilated upper pole ureter can cause secondary obstruction of the lower pole ureter. Obstruction of the upper pole system may result in a non-functioning upper pole. When the upper pole is non-functioning, renal scans and intravenous urograms give a classic appearance of the 'drooping lily'. The functioning lower pole is deviated laterally away from the spine by the large hydronephrotic upper pole. Ultrasound is useful in confirming the presence of the cystic non-functioning upper pole as the cause of the mass effect[33,34].

The ultrasonographic appearance of duplication varies, reflecting the type of duplication. In non-obstructed partial or complete duplications, the kidneys are slightly larger in size and may show a separation of the renal sinus fat. These kidneys are difficult to differentiate from kidneys with prominent columns of Bertin.

When upper pole obstruction is present, the appearance of the kidney again varies, from mild hydronephrosis involving the upper third of the kidney with a rim of normal-appearing kidney (Figure 8a,b), to hydronephrosis with thinning of

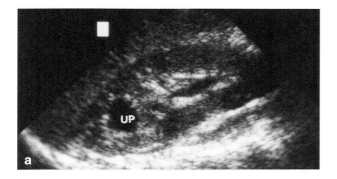

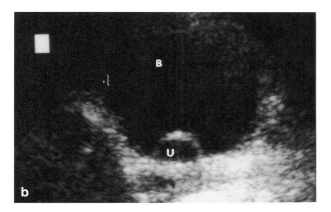

**Figure 8** (**a**) Longitudinal view of the right kidney reveals duplicated collecting system with mild hydronephrosis of both upper and lower segments (UP, upper pole renal pelvis). (**b**) Transverse view of the bladder shows a ureterocele, arising from the upper pole moiety (B, bladder; U, ureterocele)

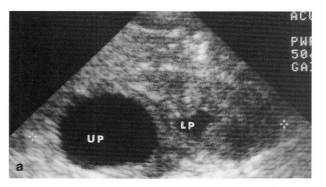

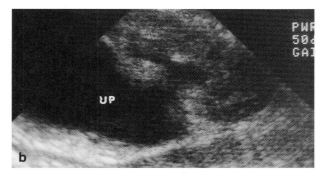

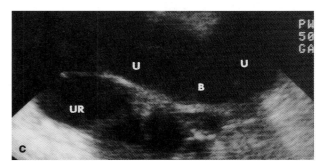

**Figure 9** (**a** – **c**) Longitudinal images of the kidneys reveal bilateral duplications with marked dilatation of the upper pole moieties and thinning of the upper pole parenchyma. The bladder is almost completely filled with two large ureteroceles. A tortuous ureter is noted behind the bladder (UP, upper pole renal pelvis; LP, lower pole renal pelvis; U, ureterocele; B, bladder; UR, ureter)

the upper pole rim parenchyma, to complete replacement of the upper third of the kidney by a large cystic mass (Figure 9). If the patient's presenting problem is a urinary tract infection or sepsis, the upper pole collecting system may contain pus and appear echogenic (Figure 10a,b,c,d). The lower pole may appear displaced from the psoas muscle by a large ectatic upper pole ureter. The ureter can often be followed to the level of the bladder. Ultrasound of the bladder is an excellent way of determining the presence of a ureterocele (Figure 11a,b,c,d). Hydronephrosis of the lower pole may be present with or without renal scarring. Voiding cystourethrography is generally used to see if the lower pole dilatation is due to reflux. This may be suggested by ultrasonography if a change in distention of the renal pelvis is noted during patient voiding. Exposure of a baby to cold gel will often result in involuntary voiding. The

bladder should therefore be evaluated early in the course of the exam[35].

## Posterior urethral valves

Posterior urethral valves are the most common cause of urethral obstruction in the male infant. Two main types are recognized. In classic posterior

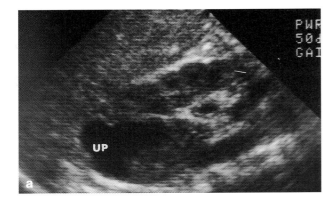

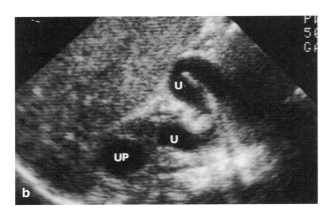

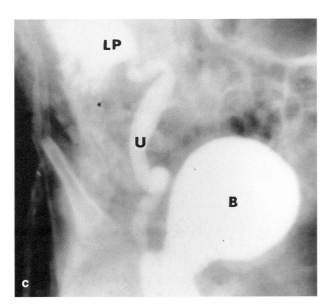

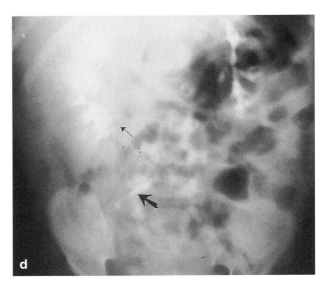

**Figure 10** (**a**) Longitudinal image of duplicated collecting system. The upper pole (UP) moiety is partially echogenic due to debris. (**b**) Transverse image showing tortuous ureter (U) and upper pole moiety (UP). (**c**) Reflux into lower pole moiety is demonstrated on a voiding cystourethrogram (B, bladder; U, ureter; LP, lower pole moiety). (**d**) Intravenous urogram showing 'drooping lily' appearance of right kidney (thin arrow) due to displacement of functioning lower pole by non-functioning upper pole. Note tortuous course of lower pole ureter as it twirls around dilated but non-visualized upper pole ureter (thick arrow)

urethral valves (type I of the Young classification), two fibro-epithelial folds of tissue originate from the lower verumontanum and extend downward and forward to insert circumferentially in the wall of the urethra. Fusion of the folds anteriorly results in a small posterior cleft as the only passageway for the urinary stream. There is associated hypertrophy of the verumontanum. The posterior urethral membrane (Young classification type III) is a less common type of valve and consists of a circumferentially attached membrane, below the level of the verumontanum at the level of the urogenital diaphragm. The veromontanum is not hypertrophied. Young described a type II valve, in which folds extend up toward the bladder neck. This type is type to be either exceedingly rare or non-existent[36,37].

Valves generally present by two years of age. They may be diagnosed in the prenatal period on ultrasound examinations done routinely or for maternal oligohydramnios (Figure 12). Identification of echogenic kidneys prenatally suggests a poor prognosis. In addition to normal echotexture, cortical renal cysts and/or hydronephrosis may be seen on both pre- and postnatal scans

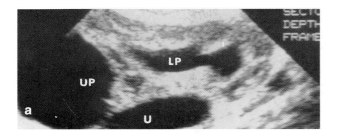

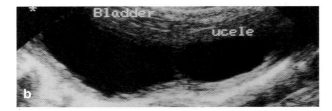

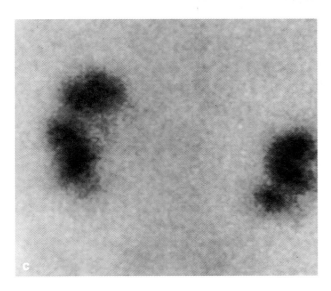

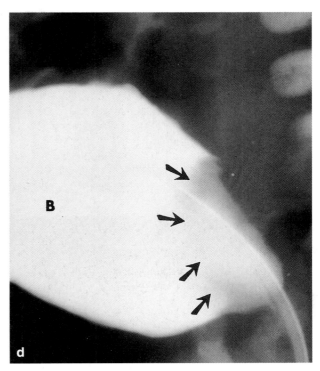

**Figure 11** (**a**) Longitudinal image of the right kidney revealing duplication with dilatation of both upper and lower pole collecting system (UP, upper pole renal pelvis; U, ureter from upper pole; LP, lower pole). (**b**) The upper pole ends in a ureterocele within the bladder. (**c**) DTPA nuclear scan on the same patient shows 'drooping lily' appearance of the right kidney due to displacement of the functioning lower pole by the non-functioning obstructed upper pole. (**d**) Voiding cystourethrogram shows a filling defect, made by a ureterocele, within the bladder (B) (outlined by arrows)

(Figure 13a,b,c,d). Hydronephrosis may be the result of obstruction or a combination of reflux and obstruction. Unilateral reflux may be present. This occasionally results in forniceal rupture and resultant urinoma formation. The function of the contralateral kidney may be preserved in these instances. The diagnosis of posterior urethral valves is classically made during voiding cysto-urethrogram (Figure 14). However, the appearance of the urinary tract in the patient with posterior urethral valves – a thick walled bladder with dilated posterior urethra – is now well described on both prenatal and postnatal ultrasound (Figure 15). Some authors advocate a transperineal approach for improved visualization of the valves[38–40].

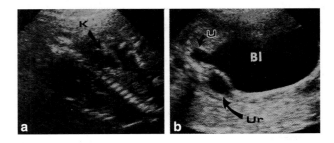

**Figure 12** (**a**), (**b**) Prenatal USG revealing dilated renal collecting systems (K) and dilated bladder (Bl), dilated ureter (Ur) and dilated urethra (U) on coronal images of the fetal abdomen (courtesy of Brian Cremin, MD, Cape Town, South Africa)

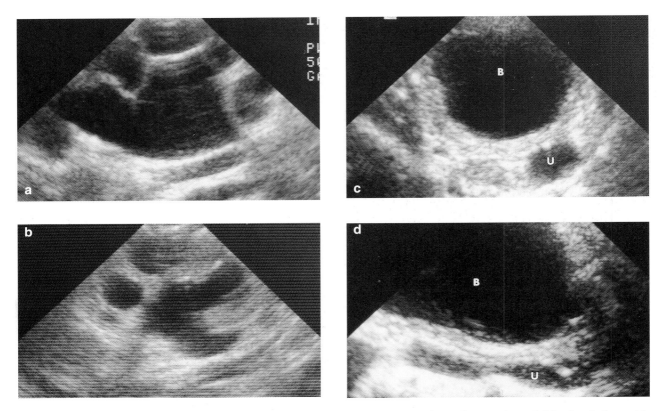

**Figure 13** (**a**) Longitudinal right kidney showing marked hydronephrosis and renal parenchymal thinning in boy with valves. (**b**) Longitudinal view of left kidney in boy with valves showing echogenic renal parenchyma and hydronephrosis. (**c**) Transverse view of thick walled bladder and dilated right ureter (B, bladder; U, ureter). (**d**) Right parasagittal view of bladder showing distended thick walled bladder and dilated ureter (B, bladder; U, ureter)

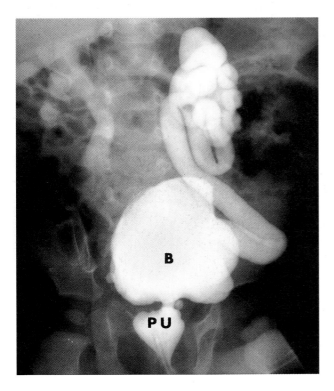

**Figure 14** (left)  Voiding cystourethrogram showing classic appearance of trabeculated bladder and dilated posterior urethra in valves (B, bladder; PU, posterior urethra)

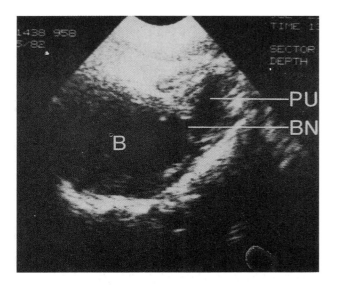

**Figure 15** Thick walled bladder (B) and dilated posterior urethra (PU) in posterior urethral valves. BN, bladder neck (courtesy of Brian Cremin, MD, Cape Town, South Africa)

## Prune belly syndrome (Eagle–Barret syndrome, Triad syndrome)

Prune belly syndrome is the triad of hypoplasia or deficiency of the abdominal musculature, cryoto-orchidism, and urinary tract anomalies. The association was first described in the 1890s. Patients demonstrate a spectrum of clinical and radiological findings (Figure 16). Most severely affected patients demonstrate urethral atresia and bilateral cystic renal dysplasia secondary to obstruction. Resultant pulmonary hypoplasia leads to neonatal death. Less severe urinary tract

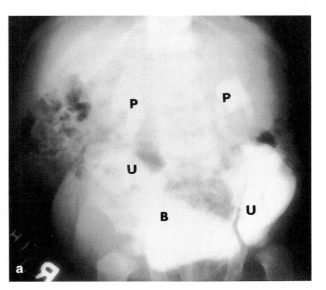

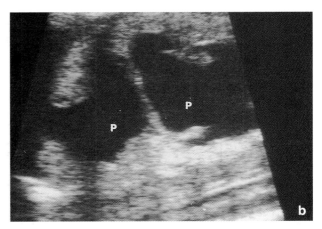

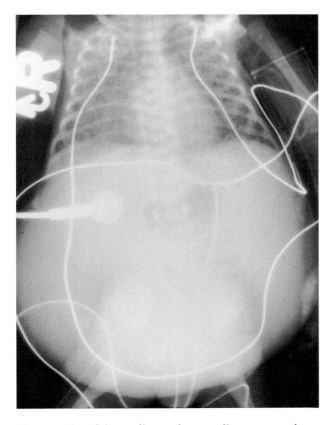

**Figure 16** Plain radiograph revealing severe lung disease and patulous abdomen due to abdominal wall musculature hypoplasia in baby with prune belly syndrome

**Figure 17** (a) Intravenous urogram showing dysplastic collecting system including misshapen kidneys and tortuous ureters (P, renal pelvis; U, ureter; B, bladder). (b) Longitudinal USG of echogenic dysplastic left kidney with dilated collecting system (P, renal pelvis)

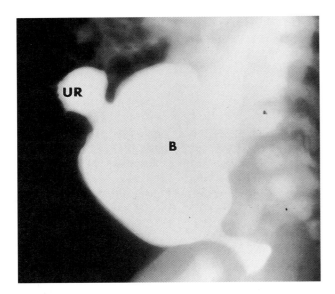

**Figure 18** Filled bladder in prune belly syndrome demonstrating urachal remnant (UR, urachal remnant; B, bladder)

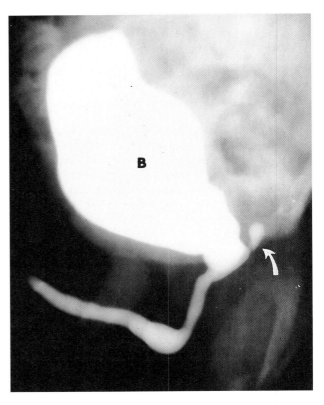

**Figure 19** Voiding cystourethrogram in prune belly syndrome demonstrating patulous bladder neck and utricle (B, bladder; arrow points to utricle)

involvement includes dilated, smooth walled bladders with poor contractility but no evidence of obstruction, oddly shaped, dysplastic kidneys, and ectactic, dilated ureters (Figure 17a,b). Though the ureters may be quite dilated, there is often no evidence of caliectasis or mechanical obstruction. Reflux is common in this syndrome. However, even in patients who do not reflux and in whom obstruction of the ureters is not demonstrated, dilatation of the ureters is commonly seen. Urachal remnants commonly arise from the dome of the bladder (Figure 18). A prominent utricle (vagina masculina) or dilated posterior urethra may be seen on voiding cystourethrography (Figure 19)[41-44].

Ultrasonographic findings vary, mirroring the clinical severity. The most severely affected babies demonstrate dysplastic echogenic kidneys[45]. Non-hydronephrotic kidneys with giant ureters and huge bladders are seen in those less severely affected. The bladder tends to be large and smooth-walled. Prenatally, the findings may be mistaken for those of posterior urethral valves. The postnatal appearance of the wrinkled prune-like abdomen makes the diagnosis much more apparent after birth.

# References

1. Haller JO, Berdon WE, Friedman AP. Increased renal cortical echogenicity: a normal finding in neonates and infants. *Radiology* 1982;142:173–4

2. Han BK, Babcock DS. Sonographic measurements and appearance of normal kidneys in children. *Am J Radiol* 1985;145:611–16

3. Hayden CK Jr, Santa-Cruz FR, Amparo EG, *et al*. Ultrasonographic evaluation of renal parenchyma in infancy and childhood. *Radiology* 1984;152:413–17

4. Hricak H, Slovis TL, Callen CW, *et al*. Neonatal kidneys: sonographic anatomic correlation. *Radiology* 1983;147:699–702

5. Shackelford GD, Kees-Folts D, Cole BR. Imaging the urinary tract. *Clin Perinatol* 1992;19:85–119

6. Brown T, Mandell J, Lebowitz RL. Neonatal hydronephrosis in the era of sonography. *Am J Radiol* 1987;148:959–63

7. Chopra A, Teele RL. Hydronephrosis in children: Narrowing the diagnosis with ultrasound. *J Clin Ultrasound* 1980;8:473–8

8. Clautice-Engle T, Anderson NG, Allan RB, et al. Diagnosis of obstructive hydronephrosis in infants: comparison sonograms performed 6 days and 6 weeks after birth. *Am J Radiol* 1995;164:963–7

9. Gill B, Levitt S, Kogan S, et al. The dilated urinary tract in children. Prospective analysis with correlation of radiological, isotope, pressure perfusion and surgical findings. *Br J Urol* 1988;61:413–19

10. Homsy Yl, Mehta PH, Huot D, et al. Intermittent hydronephrosis: a diagnostic challenge. *J Urol* 1988; 140:1222–6

11. Zerin JM. Hydronephrosis in the neonate and young infant: current concepts. *Semin US, CT, MR* 1994;15:306–16

12. Sanders RC, Hartman DS. The sonographic distinction between neonatal multicystic kidney and hydronephrosis. *Radiology* 1984;11:621–5

13. Arnold AJ, Rickwood AM. Natural history of pelviureteric obstruction detected by prenatal sonography. *Br J Urol* 1990;65:91–6

14. Fernbach SK, Maizels M, Conway JJ. Ultrasound grading of hydronephrosis: introduction to the system used by the Society for Fetal Urology. *Pediatr Radiol* 1993;23:478–80

15. Bernstein GT, Mandell J, Lebowitz RL, et al. Ureteropelvic junction obstruction in the neonate. *J Urol* 1988;140:1216–21

16. Fernbach SK, Zawin JK, Lebowitz RL. Complete duplication of the ureter with ureteropelvic junction obstruction of the lower pole of the kidney: imaging findings. *Am J Radiol* 1995;164:701–4

17. Cendron M, D'Alton ME, Crombleholme TM. Prenatal diagnosis and management of the fetus with hydronephrosis. *Semin Perinat* 1994;18:163–81

18. Dejter SW Jr, Gibbons MD. The fate of infant kidneys with fetal hydronephrosis but initially normal postnatal sonography. *J Urol* 1989;142: 661–2

19. Freedman ER, Rickwood AM. Prenatally diagnosed pelviureteric junction obstruction: a benign condition? *J Pediatr Surg* 1994;29:769–72

20. Gordon AC, Thomas DF, Arthur RJ, et al. Prenatally diagnosed reflux: a follow-up study. *Br J Urol* 1990; 65:407–12

21. Laing FC, Burke VD, Wing VW, et al. Postpartum evaluation of fetal hydronephrosis: optimal timing for follow up sonography. *Radiology* 1984;152:423–4

22. Marra G, Barbieri G, Moioli C, et al. Mild fetal hydronephrosis indicating vesicoureteric reflux. *Arch Dis Child Fetal Neonat Edn* 1994;70:147–50

23. Maizels M, Mitchell B, Kass E, et al. Outcome of nonspecific hydronephrosis in the infant: a report from the registry of the Society for Fetal Urology. *J Urol* 1994;152:2324–7

24. Ransley PG, Dhillion HK, Gordon I, et al. The postnatal management of hydronephrosis diagnosed by prenatal ultrasound. *J Urol* 1990;22: 379–81

25. Tam JC, Hodson EM, Choong KK, et al. Postnatal diagnosis and outcome of urinary tract abnormalities detected by antenatal ultrasound. *Med J Austral* 1994;160:633–7

26. Zerin JM, Ritchey MI, Chang AC. Incidental vesicoureteral reflux in neonates with antenatally detected hydronephrosis and other renal abnormalities. *Radiology* 1993;187:157–60

27. Meyer JS, Lebowitz RL. Primary megaureter in infants and children: a review. *Urol Radiol* 1992;14: 296–305

28. Wood BP, Ben-Ami T, Teele RL, et al. Ureterovesical obstruction and megaloureter. Diagnosis by real-time US. *Radiology* 1985;156:79–81

29. Nussbaum AR, Dorst JP, Jeffs RD, et al. Ectopic ureter and ureterocele: their varied sonographic manifestations. *Radiology* 1986;159:227–35

30. Kessler RM, Altman DH. Real-time sonographic detection of vesicoureteral reflux in children. *Am J Radiol* 1982;138:1033–6

31. Paltiel HJ, Lebowitz RL. Neonatal hydronephrosis due to primary vesicoureteral reflux: trends in diagnosis and treatment. *Radiology* 1989;170:787–9

32. Schneider K, Jablonski C, Weissner M, et al. Screening for vesicoureteral reflux in children using real-time sonography. *Pediatr Radiol* 1984;14:400–3

33. Horgan JG, Rosenfield NS, Weiss RM, et al. Is renal ultrasound a reliable indicator of a nonobstructed duplication anomaly? *Pediatr Radiol* 1984;14:388–91

34. Schaffer RM, Shih YH, Becker JA. Sonographic identification of collecting system duplications. *J Clin Ultrasound* 1983;11:309–12

35. Athey PA, Carpenter RJ, Hadlock RP, et al. Ultrasonic demonstration of ectopic ureterocele. *Pediatrics* 1983;71:568–71

36. Cohen HL, Susman M, Haller JO, et al. Posterior urethral valve; transperineal US for imaging and diagnostic evaluation. *Radiology* 1994;192:261–4

37. Cremin BJ, Aaronson IA. Ultrasonic diagnosis of posterior urethral valve in neonates. *Br J Radiol* 1983;56:435–8

38. Macpherson RI, Leithiser RE, Gordon L, et al. Posterior urethral valves: an update and review. *Radiographics* 1986;6:753–91

39. McAlister WH. Demonstration of the dilated prostatic urethra in posterior urethral valves patients. *J Ultrasound Med* 1984;3:189–90

40. Rittenberg MH, Hurlbert WC, Snyder HM III, et al. Protective features in posterior urethral valves. *J Urol* 1988;140:993–6

41. Berdon WE, Baker DH, Wigger HJ, *et al*. The radiologic and pathologic spectrum of the prune belly syndrome. *Radiol Clin North Am* 1977;15: 83–92

42. Burbige KA, Amodio J, Berdon WE, *et al*. Prune belly syndrome: 35 years of experience. *J Urol* 1987; 137:86–90

43. Garris J, Kangerloo H, Sarti D, *et al*. The ultrasound spectrum of prune belly syndrome. *J Clin Ultrasound* 1980;8:117–20

44. Fernbach SK. The dilated urinary tract in children. *Urol Radiol* 1992;14:34–42

45. Sanders RC, Nussbaum AR, Solez K. Renal dysplasia; sonographic findings. *Radiology* 1988;167:623–6

# Sonography of the neonatal ovary

9

*Sandra Schmahmann and Jack O. Haller*

This chapter reviews the literature with an emphasis on sonographic findings of the normal neonatal ovary, neonatal ovarian cyst, neonatal ovarian torsion, and ovarian teratoma in the neonate and young female.

## The normal neonatal ovary

Follicular growth and development in the ovary is a dynamic, continuous process which begins in the fetus and continues during childhood. Neonatal ovaries are similar in function and anatomy to pubertal and adult ovaries. Oocytes, as well as differentiating and maturing follicles, co-exist in the neonatal ovary. The mean number of follicles is 266 000, the majority of which are primordial, with the remainder being primary, secondary, and Graafian. The cortex forms four-fifths of the neonatal ovary, which has a mean volume of 126 mm³. The neonatal ovarian volume is comprised of interstitium (35–40%), medulla with blood vessels and nerves (10–30%), and follicles (10–25%)[1].

Key sonographic studies of ovaries in children from the mid-1980s describe the typical ovary as homogeneous in echogenicity, with cysts being an uncommon finding, particularly in children less than six years old[2].

With improvement in sonographic technology, ovarian cysts have been found in the majority of neonatal and infant ovaries. Cohen *et al.* described the morphology and volume of normal ovaries in girls one day to two months old[3]. The typical neonatal and infant ovary was found to be heterogeneous and cystic. In patients aged between one day and three months, cysts of less than 9 mm were noted in 82% of imaged ovaries, macrocysts (larger than 9 mm) were seen in 20% of the cystic ovaries. The mean diameter of the largest cyst of each ovary was 7.5 mm. The mean ovarian volume of this age group was 1.06 cm³ [3].

In 1861, Rokitansky stated in the pathology literature that cystic follicles may be seen in the ovaries of fetuses, neonates, and children[2]. Polhemus also found that extensive follicular growth is normal during childhood and observed that ovarian follicles begin maturing at or before birth[2].

Ovarian cysts develop from ovarian follicles. Size is the primary difference between a pathological cyst and physiological mature follicle. Cysts larger than 2 cm are considered to be pathological[4].

Follicle-stimulating hormone (FSH), maternal estrogens, and human chorionic gonadotropin (hCG) all contribute to follicular growth *in utero*. However, the primary stimulus is FSH, which is secreted by the fetal pituitary and which increases both the number and size of individual follicles. The hormonal balance present during the last months of fetal life contributes to further follicular growth.

At birth, maternal estrogens and hCG levels fall with the separation of the placenta from the neonate. FSH levels decline as a result of the inhibitory mechanism of the hypothalamus pituitary ovary axis.

FSH production is inhibited in the full-term infant by even very low levels of circulatory estrogens, gradually decreasing the FSH level during the first year of life. The premature infant with an immature gonadostat may produce FSH for a longer period[3,4].

## Neonatal ovarian cysts

### Etiology

Although the etiology of neonatal cysts is unclear, it is likely that they result from disordered folliculogenesis occurring in the fetal ovary[5]. Fetal ovarian cysts usually resolve spontaneously, but they may persist into the neonatal period.

The presence of small follicular cysts of 3–7 mm is a common and normal finding in neonatal ovaries. De Sa, in an autopsy study, showed small follicular cysts in 34% of still births and neonates within the first 28 days of life[1,6,7]. Neonatal ovarian cysts are primarily of follicular origin. The types of cysts identified in pathologic study include simple, follicular, corpus luteum, and theca lutein cysts[1,7,8]. Evidence suggests that excessive stimulation of the fetal ovary by both placental and maternal hormones may be a significant factor in cyst development[4,5,7]. There is an increased incidence of cysts in infants of mothers with diabetes, toxemia, or rhesus immunization presumably from hypersecretion of placental hCG or increased placental permeability to hCG[1,7,9,10].

Follicular cysts have been described in maternal and congenital hypothyroidism. Non-specific pituitary glycoprotein hormone synthesis has been cited as the explanation for the follicular cysts seen in patients with longstanding juvenile hypothyroidism[1,11,12].

The functional origin of these ovarian cysts is confirmed by the presence of high levels of estradiol, progesterone, and testosterone found within the majority of the cysts[5].

## Complications

Neonatal ovarian cysts frequently regress spontaneously and rarely cause severe symptoms[1,4,12,13]. The complications that do occur are divided into primary, secondary, and maternal sequelae[1].

Salpingotorsion and hemorrhage are the most frequent primary complications. Torsion is more common in large cysts, but has been reported in cysts as small as 2 cm[1,4,7,10]. Mulle-Leisse *et al.*, in a large study of 49 cysts, reported that torsion occurred in 42% of patients. This result corresponds with other series, including that of Nussbaum *et al.*[7,10]. The reported incidence of torsion has been as high as 50–78%. These torsions, many of which occur antenatally[4,7], may be accompanied by pain, vomiting, fever, abdominal distention, leukocytosis, and peritonitis. However, many cases are asymptomatic[7,10].

Hemorrhage into a cyst may result from torsion or occur in a non-twisted cyst. Most authors have found that hemorrhagic cysts almost uniformly result from torsion and associated infarction, whereas others believe that mechanical stress during delivery causes hemorrhage[7,10]. A potentially lethal, but rare, complication is cyst rupture causing hemorrhagic ascites, and/or peritonitis[1,7].

Secondary complications from large cysts include bowel obstruction, thorax compression (with pulmonary hypoplasia), urinary tract obstruction or incarceration within an inguinal hernia[1,4,7,9].

Polyhydramnios and vaginal dystocia are the rare maternal complications of fetal ovarian cysts[1,7]. Polyhydramnios has been reported in 5–12% of cases[7]. Two theories regarding the etiology of polyhydramnios are partial obstruction of the small bowel and compression of the umbilical cord[7,11]. Large cysts of 12 and 19 cm have been associated with dystocia and cyst rupture[7].

## Sonographic appearance

There is a great variation in the size of ovarian cysts ranging from 1.5–19 cm. The larger cysts may occupy almost the entire abdomen[4,7,8,9,12,14] (Figure 1).

The appearance of a cyst varies, depending on whether the cyst is uncomplicated or complicated by torsion or hemorrhage. An uncomplicated cyst is anechoic with an imperceptible wall. A complicated cyst invariably contains a fluid-debris level, a retracting clot, septa, or may be completely filled with echoes producing a solid mass-like appearance (Figure 2a,b). These complex cysts often have echogenic walls resulting from dystrophic calcification associated with infarction[7,10].

In Nussbaum's study, a fluid debris level and retracting clot were found to be specific signs of torsion which had occurred before birth in the majority of cases[7]. In Mulle-Leisse's study, uncomplicated cysts developed intraluminal echoes of varying morphology postnatally, which the authors attributed to mechanical stress of delivery and not to torsion[10]. Nussbaum also found that the ovary contralateral to an ovarian cyst is frequently multi-cystic[7].

## Differential diagnosis

It may be impossible to differentiate an ovarian cyst from a mesenteric or enteric cyst[7,8,10,15]. Enteric duplication cysts have been described by Barr *et al.*

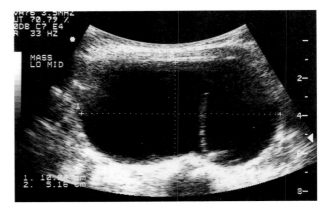

**Figure 1** Longitudinal scan of the pelvis in the midline shows a large simple cystic mass with one septation. The mass, an ovarian cyst, occupies the entire abdominal cavity

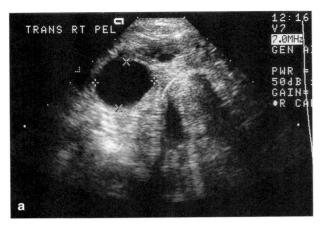

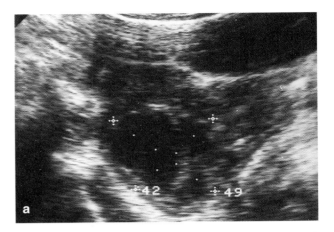

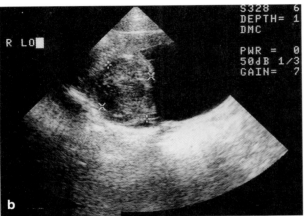

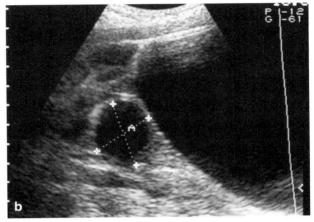

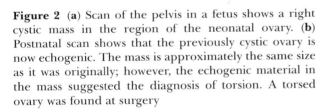

**Figure 2** (a) Scan of the pelvis in a fetus shows a right cystic mass in the region of the neonatal ovary. (b) Postnatal scan shows that the previously cystic ovary is now echogenic. The mass is approximately the same size as it was originally; however, the echogenic material in the mass suggested the diagnosis of torsion. A torsed ovary was found at surgery

**Figure 3** (a) Longitudinal scan of the pelvis shows a left adnexal mass with cystic and solid components. (b) Two weeks later the mass had decreased in size and appeared as a simple cyst; the diagnosis of hemorrhagic ovarian cyst was made

as having a hyperechoic mucosal layer with an underlying hypoechoic layer in all cases[16].

Other cystic structures which may be confused with ovarian cysts are hydrometrocolpos, cystic meconium peritonitis, urachal cyst, bowel atresia or obstruction, renal cysts, and anterior meningocoele[1,7,8,10,15,17].

Complex cysts, especially those presenting as a solid mass or a cystic mass with a retracting clot, may be impossible to differentiate from a neoplasm (Figure 3a,b). Ovarian neonatal neoplasms are extremely rare, and include cystadenomas, cystic teratomas, and granulosa cell tumors[4,7,8,17].

## Management

The management options for treating a neonatal ovarian cyst largely depend upon cyst size and sonographic characteristics. Other factors involved are the potential risk of complications and the differentiation of ovarian cysts from other ovarian tumors and from other intraperitoneal cystic masses[4,8].

After birth, the decrease in hormonal stimulation which occurs is associated with spontaneous regression of most small cysts. Therefore, ovarian cyst formation in the perinatal period is a self-limiting process. Simple ovarian cysts which are less than 4 cm can thus be safely observed, and their resolution followed, using serial ultrasonography. Most cysts will resolve in three to four months, but longer periods of observation may be necessary if the cyst is decreasing in size[4,8].

The treatment of larger cysts and complex cysts remains controversial[4,7,8,9,17]. Cysts larger than 4 cm are associated with a greater risk of torsion. Because ovarian torsion may lead to loss of the ovary, early intervention may be required. The management options include surgery, needle aspiration, or laparoscopy. When surgery is performed, it is important to preserve as much gonadal tissue as possible and merely remove or unroof the cyst. Ovarian cysts are often adherent to the ovary and many times oophorectomy cannot be avoided[4,8]. Ultrasound-guided needle aspiration of the cyst has no reported complications and offers excellent possibilities with respect to preserving the ovary[4].

Successful laparoscopic approach to the management of ovarian cysts has been reported. This technique appears to be promising and offers both diagnostic capabilities (visualization and biopsy) as well as smooth transition to therapeutic measures, when necessary. Cysts can be decapsulated by use of a laser or surgical incision, thus saving the ovary[18].

## Ovarian torsion

Torsion of the ovary can occur at any age and, although it is rare in the infant, there are reported cases of neonatal ovarian torsion[19,20].

Torsion of normal ovaries usually occurs in the first two decades of life. The normal adnexa in girls may be very mobile, allowing torsion at the mesosalpinx with changes in intra-abdominal pressure or body position[21]. Although ovarian torsion can occur in normal ovaries, it is more common in cases of ovarian cysts and tumors. The enlarged pathological ovary acts as a fulcrum potentiating torsion of the ovary and fallopian tubes[21,22].

Adults and children with ovarian torsion usually have clinical symptoms of severe abdominal pain, which leads to surgical exploration and subsequent removal of the ovary[19,22,23]. In infants, more commonly than adults, the torsion may be missed clinically, because there are no symptoms or non-specific symptoms[19]. The ovary and fallopian tube then undergo necrosis and amputation. The amputated ovary may resorb completely which results in an absent ovary; however, it is more common for the ovary to detach completely and become a loose calcified fibrotic nodule which moves freely in the peritoneal cavity, often in the cul-de-sac[19,24].

Sonography is valuable in establishing the diagnosis of ovarian torsion, and in excluding other causes of acute lower abdominal pain, such as appendicitis, gastroenteritis, pyelonephritis, or pelvic inflammatory disease[21,22].

Stark and Siegel studied the sonographic findings of ovarian torsion in prepubertal and pubertal girls, and concluded that there are differences between the two age groups. Color Doppler imaging, however, was not decisive. Arterial perfusion was found to be variable and color Doppler waveforms were seen in both groups[25]. Gray scale sonographic findings were more specific. While both groups had enlarged ovaries, the location and appearance of the twisted ovaries varied. In the older child and adolescent the masses were adnexal, while in the neonate and infant they were extrapelvic (Figures 4a,b,c and 5a,b). In all neonates and several infants complex masses with multiple large cysts, septations, and debris levels were observed. Pubertal girls tended to have enlarged solid ovaries, often with cortically based cysts[25].

Fluid in the cul-de-sac has been reported as a late manifestation of ovarian torsion and usually represents non-viability of the ovary[23].

In cases of ovarian torsion and amputation, the ovary detaches from the adnexa and migrates to other sites in the abdomen, parasitizing vascular supply. These cysts are pedunculated and the pedicle consists of mesentery and omentum. The mass is therefore located in variable positions in the abdomen, and mobility of these calcified masses can be documented on radiographs. The nature of the calcifications has no distinguishing characteristics of differential value. Sonography reveals a cystic mass containing a solid partially calcified mural nodule[19,24].

No clearly recognizable ovarian tissues have been reported in the majority of amputated ovaries. It is thought that the original ovaries were probably normal, and the cystic and calcified nature of the mass represents sequelae of necrosis and hemorrhage (Figure 6). It is not possible to exclude that an ovarian cyst or possibly a teratoma was present in the ovary prior to this torsion and amputation[19,24].

## Ovarian teratomas

Ovarian enlargement in the neonate is largely due to non-neoplastic cysts. There are several ovarian neoplasms that have been reported in the neonatal period including two ovarian teratomas. Three cystadenomas and three granulosa cell tumors have also been described[4,7,26,27].

Ovarian tumors are uncommon in the child and adolescent. Germ cell tumors account for 60% of ovarian neoplasms in patients less than 20 years of age, which differs from the situation in adults, in

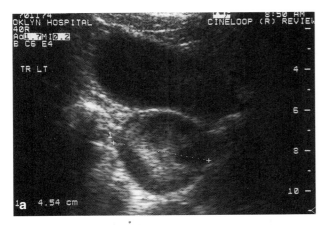

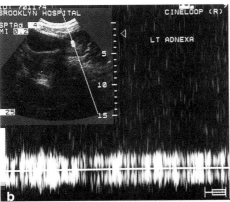

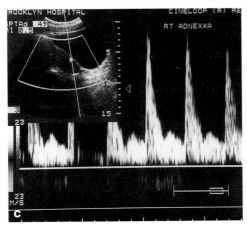

**Figure 4** (a) Longitudinal scan of the left ovary shows an enlarged edematous ovary with hypoechoic rim. The mass was palpable and was accompanied by laboratory findings of an increased white blood cell count. The child was irritable and in pain. (b) and (c) Doppler studies of the left and right ovaries, respectively, show significant flow in the right ovary as compared with the left. While the latter is not diagnostic it was corroborative of the clinical suspicions. A torsed ovary was removed at surgery

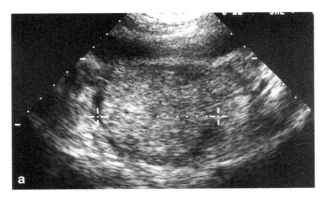

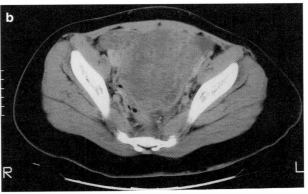

**Figure 5** (a) Transverse sonogram of the pelvis shows an enlarged echogenic mass with a slight hypoechoic rim. The mass extended outside the pelvis and was felt in the mid-abdomen. (b) CT scan of the upper pelvis shows a mixed attenuation mass occupying virtually the entire pelvis. This was a 10-year-old girl and the mass upon removal proved to be an ovarian torsion

whom 20% of ovarian tumors are of germ cell origin, and in whom epithelial tumors predominate[26,28,29].

Norris and Jensen studied the relative frequency of ovarian neoplasms in children and adolescents, and their relationship to the age of the patient. They reported that the highest incidence of germ cell tumors occurred in children between the ages of 10–14 years. The 5–9 year olds represented the next group, followed by children aged 15–19 years and lastly by children less than 4 years[28,29] (Figure 7a,b,c).

There is a spectrum of germ cell tumors ranging from the benign mature teratomas through the malignant varieties, which are the dysgerminomas, embryonal carcinomas, endodermal sinus tumors, immature teratomas, choriocarcinomas, and mixed tumors[26,28]. The benign mature teratoma or dermoid cyst is by far the most common pediatric germ cell tumor, and accounts for approximately 30–50% of these neoplasms[26,28,29].

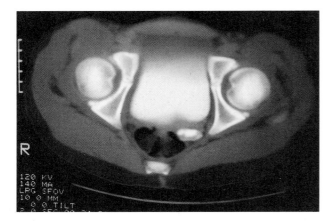

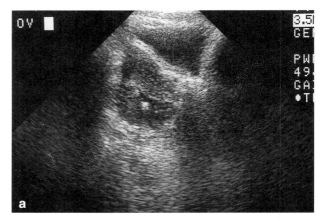

**Figure 6** CT scan of the pelvis for other reasons showed an incidental calcific density behind the left side of the bladder and anterior to the rectum. On exploration the left ovary was not present. The mass was diagnosed as previously calcified torsed and amputated left ovary

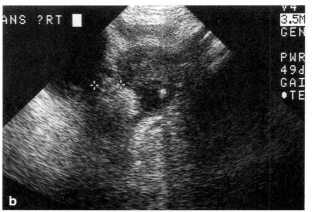

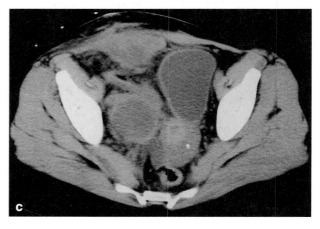

Mature teratomas are made up of a variety of tissues reflecting their pluripotential germ cell origin. A central cystic cavity filled with sebaceous debris is surrounded by a variety of skin appendages, a squamous epithelial layer, and a thick capsule. A nubbin of tissue also referred to as a dermal plug or mural nodule is frequently found in the wall of a teratoma. This nodule often contains all three germ cell layers. Most dermoid cysts are between 5 and 15 cm in size, however they can range from 3 to 23 cm[26,28,30].

It is interesting that there is a difference in the bilaterality of teratomas in adults versus children. Twenty-five per cent of teratomas occur bilaterally in adults, compared with a lower incidence of 0–10% in children[26,28,30,31]. No explanation can be found for this difference in bilaterality. Perhaps, when pediatric germ cell tumors are diagnosed, if there is involvement of the contralateral ovary the germ cell tumor is too small to be detected.

The majority of dermoids are asymptomatic. When there are symptoms the patient most commonly presents with abdominal pain or may have a palpable abdominal or pelvic mass[26,28,30]. The diagnosis of teratomas is incidental in approximately half of the cases, either during unrelated surgery or following abdominal radiographs. Most series indicate that 50% of dermoids show radiological evidence of their presence in the form of ossification or teeth. All varieties of teeth can be found, although incisors are less frequently seen. The finding of recognizable teeth in the pelvis essentially makes the diagnosis of a teratoma[26–28,32].

**Figure 7** (a) and (b) Longitudinal and transverse scans respectively of the pelvis in a 9-month-old girl show a mass behind the uterus. The mass has a focus of increased echogenicity with shadowing. The mass is surrounded by low level echoes as well. (c) Transverse scan shows the mass to be anterior to the rectum and posterior to the bladder, and contain a speck of calcium. An ovarian teratoma tumor was removed at surgery

The most frequent complication of teratoma is torsion, which occurs in 16–40% of cases. Abdominal pain is the most common complaint. If the dermoid cyst is on the right side, the pain may mimic acute appendicitis. Surgical removal of the ovary is usually performed when torsion is found[26,28].

Rupture or perforation of the dermoid cyst is very rare and occurs in less than 1% of patients. Generalized peritonitis occurs when the cyst ruptures, resulting in a surgical emergency, necessitating irrigation and removal of the contents of the cyst[28].

Teratomas can be detected easily by sonography because of their large size. Although easily recognizable, their appearance is often non-specific and variable because of their heterogeneous composition[30]. Mural nodules and echogenic foci with acoustic shadowing are the typical findings on ultrasound[30]. Sisler and Siegel compared the sonographic appearance of ovarian teratomas in prepubertal and postpubertal girls. Both acoustic shadowing and mural nodules were more frequently seen in postpubertal girls. Microscopic calcifications not large enough to produce shadowing, or calcifications hidden within matted hair, were given as possible explanations for the lower incidence of acoustic shadowing in prepubertal girls. The reason that mural nodules were seen less often in prepubertal girls was attributed to the small size (< 5 mm) of the nodules[30].

It is important to preserve fertility and ovarian function in these young patients. The treatment of dermoid cysts involves resection of the cyst from the ovary, attempting to conserve as much ovarian tissue as possible[28].

# References

1. Kurjak A. *Ultrasound and the Ovary*. Carnforth, UK: Parthenon Publishing, 1994:7,59,33–44
2. Cohen HL, Eisenberg P, Mandel F, *et al.* Ovarian cysts are common in premenarchal girls. A sonographic study of 101 children 2–12 years old. *Am J Roentgenol* 1992;159:89–91
3. Cohen HL, Shapiro MA, Mandel FS, *et al.* Normal ovaries in neonates and infants. A sonographic study of 77 patients 1 day–24 months old. *Am J Roentgenol* 1993;160:583–6
4. Brandt ML, Luks FI, Filiatrault D, *et al.* Surgical indications in antenatally diagnosed ovarian cysts. *J Pediatr Surg* 1991;26:276–82
5. Montag TW, Auletta FW, Gibson M. Neonatal ovarian cyst: prenatal diagnosis and analysis of the cyst fluid. *Obstet Gynecol* 1983;61:38–41
6. De Sa DJ. Follicular ovarian cysts in stillbirths and neonates. *Arch Dis Child* 1975;50:45–50
7. Nussbaum AR, Sanders RC, Hartman DS, *et al.* Neonatal ovarian cysts: sonographic-pathologic correlation. *Radiology* 1988;168:817–21
8. Garel L, Filiatrault D, Brandt M, *et al.* Antenatal diagnosis of ovarian cysts: natural history and therapeutic implications. *Pediatr Radiol* 1991;21:182–4
9. Nussbaum AR, Sanders RC, Benator RM, *et al.* Spontaneous resolution of neonatal ovarian cysts. *Am J Roentgenol* 1987;148:175–6
10. Muller-Leisse C, Bick U, Paullussen K, *et al.* Ovarian cysts in the fetus and neonate – changes in sonographic pattern in their follow-up and management. *Pediatr Radiol* 1992;22:395–400
11. Jafri SZH, Bree RL, Silver TM, *et al.* Fetal ovarian cysts: sonographic detection and association with hypothyroidism. *Radiology* 1984;150:809–12
12. Meizner J, Levy A, Katz M, *et al.* Fetal ovarian cysts: prenatal ultrasonographic detection and postnatal evaluation and treatment. *J Obstet Gynecol* 1991;164:874–8
13. Suita S, Ikeda K, Koyanagi T, *et al.* Neonatal ovarian cyst diagnosed antenatally: report of two patients. *J Clin Ultrasound* 1991;12:517–19
14. Bagolan P, Rivosecchi M, Giorlandino C, *et al.* Prenatal diagnosis and clinical outcome of ovarian cysts. *J Pediatr Surg* 1992;27:879–81
15. Haller JO, Schneider M, Kassner EG, *et al.* Sonographic evaluation of mesenteric and omental masses in children. *Am J Roentgenol* 1978;130:269–74
16. Barr LL, Hayden CK Jr, Stansberry SD, *et al.* Enteric duplication cysts in children: are their ultrasonographic wall characteristics diagnostic? *Pediatr Radiol* 1990;20:326
17. Croitoru DP, Aaron LE, Laberge JM, *et al.* Management of complex ovarian cysts presenting in the first year of life. *J Pediatr Surg* 1991;26:1366–8
18. Van der Zee DC, van Seumeren IGC, Bax KMA, *et al.* Laparoscopic approach to surgical management of ovarian cysts in the newborn. *J Pediatr Surg* 1995;30:42–3
19. Currarino G, Rutledge JC. Ovarian torsion and amputation resulting in partially calcified pedunculated cystic mass. *Pediatr Radiol* 1989;19:395–9
20. Alrabee A, Galliani CA, Giacomantino M, *et al.* Neonatal ovarian torsion: report of three cases and a review of the literature. *Pediatr Pathol* 1988;8:143–9
21. Farrel TP, Boal DK, Teele RL, *et al.* Acute torsion of normal uterine adnexa in children: sonographic demonstration. *Am J Radiol* 1982;139:1223–5

22. Graif M, Itzchak Y. Sonographic evaluation of ovarian torsion in childhood and adolescence. *Am J Radiol* 1988;150:647–9

23. Worthington-Kirsch RL, Raptopolous V, Cohen IT. Sequential bilateral torsion of normal ovaries in a child. *J Ultrasound Med* 1986;5:663–4

24. Kennedy LA, Pinckney LE, Currarino G, *et al.* Amputated calcified ovaries in children. *Radiology* 1981;141:83–6

25. Stark JE, Siegel MJ. Ovarian torsion in prepubertal and postpubertal girls: sonographic findings. *Am J Radiol* 1994;163:1479–82

26. Breen JL, Maxson WS. Ovarian tumors in children and adolescents. *Clin Obstet Gynecol* 1977;20:607–22

27. Marshall JR. Ovarian enlargement in the first year of life. *Ann Surg* 1965;161:372–7

28. Jones HW, Wentz AC, Burnett LS *Novak's Textbook of Gynecology.* Baltimore, MD: Williams and Wilkins, 1988:831–47

29. Norris HJ, Jensen RD. Relative frequency of ovarian neoplasms in children and adolescents. *Cancer* 1972;30:713–18

30. Sisler CL, Siegel MJ. Ovarian teratomas: a comparison of the sonographic appearance in pre-pubertal and postpubertal girls. *Am J Radiol* 1989; 154:139–42

31. Siegel MJ, McAlister WH, Shackelford GD. Radiographic findings in ovarian teratomas in children. *Am J Radiol* 1978;131:613–16

32. Abell MR, Johnson VJ. Ovarian neoplasms in childhood and adolescence 1. Tumors of germ cell origin. *Am J Obstet Gynecol* 1965;92:1059–81

# Developmental displacement of the neonatal hip

## 10

*Michael A. Cook*

There are several indications for sonography of the neonatal hip. The most common indication is the evaluation of the neonate thought to have developmental displacement of the hip. Other indications include septic arthritis to exclude a joint effusion and in the evaluation of patients thought to have proximal focal femoral deficiency.

## Dislocation of the hip

There are several types of dislocated hips seen in the pediatric population: acquired, teratogenic, and developmental. Acquired causes of hip dislocation include traumatic and non-traumatic etiologies (i.e. neuromuscular diseases). Teratogenic dislocations occur *in utero* and are associated with neuromuscular disorders. Developmental dislocation of the hip was formerly known as 'congenital hip dysplasia'. Since the term 'congenital hip dysplasia' includes a wide spectrum of pathology and usually occurs after birth it has been replaced by the term 'developmental displacement of the hip' (DDH). This is a broader term which includes dysplastic, subluxated, dislocatable, and dislocated hips[1].

## Developmental displacement of the hip

Developmental displacement of the hip is a relatively common congenital abnormality which can be diagnosed in the neonatal period. Plain film radiographs have historically been used to confirm the diagnosis in neonates suspected of having DDH on clinical examination. Sonography has emerged as the preferred screening and diagnostic imaging modality since it does not require sedation, provides excellent soft tissue differentiation, and does not involve ionizing radiation and can therefore be repeated safely[2]. Sonography has also been found to be more sensitive than physical examination in the detection of DDH[3,4].

## Epidemiology

The overall incidence of DDH is between 0.3 and 4 per 1000 live births[5,6]. There are several risk factors which are associated with DDH[5,6] (Table 1). Most cases occur in the first born child and females outnumber males by 8 : 1[5]. The left hip (11 : 1) is more commonly affected than the right[5]. Approximately 5% of the cases are bilateral[5]. Whites are more commonly affected than Blacks[5]. The incidence of DDH may be marginally higher in children born by cesarian section and is more common in those children born breech[7]. Very low birth weight (<1500 g) has not been shown to be a risk factor[8]. Other reported risk factors include maternal hypertension, fetal growth retardation, oligohydramnios, premature rupture of membranes, prolonged gestation, increased birth weight, Potter's syndrome and neonatal intensive care[8,9].

Associated anomalies include congenital torticollis, metatarsus adductus, calcaneovalgus feet, spina bifida, and sacral dimples[6,9]. Teratogenic dislocations are associated with arthrogryposis and myelodysplasia and are irreducible[9].

## Etiology

The primary cause of DDH is uncertain but is thought to be due to ligamentous laxity around the hip joint[6]. Genetic, mechanical, and physiological factors are thought to play a role.

Genetic factors are implicated because there is a 6% chance that a child will be affected if a sibling has DDH and a 36% chance if one sibling and one parent are affected. There is a 12% chance that an affected individual will have a child with DDH[6]. Developmental dysplasia of the hip has been associated with HLA–DR4 antigens[10].

Mechanical causes are thought to play a role since oligohydramnios, breech presentation, and the primigravid uterus are risk factors. In each case, mobility of the hip is limited. Oligohydramnios limits mobility because there is less than a

**Table 1**    Risk factors for developmental displacement of the hip

Primigravid uterus
Positive family history
Female child
Breech presentation
White child
Oligohydramnios

normal amount of amniotic fluid which makes the amniotic cavity small. In breech presentation the fetus's hip (usually the left) rests against the maternal sacrum and is usually flexed which limits movement. The frank breech position in which the hips are maximally flexed and the knees are extended carries the highest risk. The primigravid uterus is smaller than the multigravid uterus and is therefore more confining and limits mobility.

Maternal estrogen might play a physiological role by blocking the maturation of collagen and thereby promoting ligamentous laxity. However, this is unproven.

## Physical examination

The diagnosis of DDH depends on careful physical examination[11]. Visual inspection demonstrates the dislocated hip to have asymmetric skin folds and shortening of the affected thigh. The knee is also lower in position on the affected side when the patient is supine and the knees are flexed (Galaezzi's sign).

There are two basic maneuvers which are helpful in the diagnosis of DDH. The Barlow maneuver determines if the hip can be dislocated. This maneuver is performed by having the patient lie in the supine position with the hip flexed 90° and adducted. Downward and outward pressure is then applied. If the hip can be dislocated the examiner will feel the femoral head move out of the acetabulum with his fingers. The Ortolani maneuver determines if the dislocated femoral head can be reduced back into the acetabulum. The patient lies in the supine position. The examiner's hand is placed around the hip to be examined, with the fingers over the femoral head. The examiner's middle finger lies over the greater trochanter and the thumb is over the lesser trochanter. The hip is flexed 90° and the thigh is abducted. Movement in the normal hip should feel smooth. In cases of DDH, a 'clunk' is appreciated as the femoral head returns into the acetabulum. A

'click' does not imply DDH. Each hip should be examined individually.

## Imaging strategies

Multiple modalities are available to diagnose and manage DDH. The diagnosis can be established with radiography, computed tomography (CT), magnetic resonance imaging (MRI) and sonography[12,13]. Radiography is not the ideal screening or diagnostic modality since it utilizes ionizing radiation and is not able to visualize the soft tissue components of the hip or the unossified femoral head nucleus. Radiography is not useful before four to six months of age due to lack of bony changes. CT and MRI are not ideal screening or diagnostic modalities since they are expensive and may require sedation. CT also involves ionizing radiation. Sonography is the ideal screening and diagnostic modality because it does not require sedation, provides very good soft tissue differentiation, does not utilize ionizing radiation, and can be performed through a cast, brace or harness. CT and MRI can be used to check the position of the femoral head in relation to the acetabulum in patients who undergo treatment. MRI is also helpful in patients who present late, are thought to have a complex dislocation and when complications such as avascular necrosis are suspected[14]. Arthrography is invasive but useful in complicated cases which present late or when treatment fails.

### Radiography

The radiographic diagnosis of DDH has traditionally been made with a supine radiograph of the pelvis with the hips in neutral position. The diagnosis required a series of lines to be drawn and measurements made on the image[6] (Figure 1). Hilgenreiner's line is a horizontal line drawn through the triradiate cartilage. Perkin's line is a vertical line drawn down from the lateral rim of the acetabulum. The intersection of Hilgenreiner's and Perkin's line creates four quadrants in the hip. The femoral head should lie within the lower inner quadrant. If the femoral head does not fall within this quadrant the hip is dislocated. Shenton's line is a curvilinear line drawn along the medial border of the femur and along the superior border of the obturator foramen. This line should be smooth and continuous. If it is not smooth and continuous the hip is dislocated. The acetabular angle or

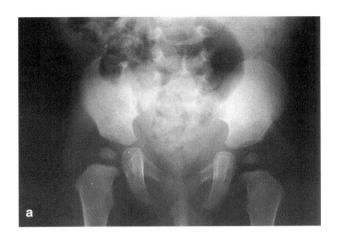

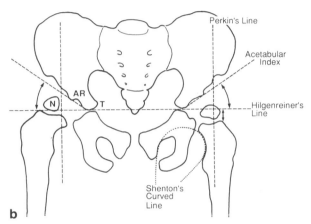

**Figure 1** Radiographic evaluation of developmental dysplasia of the hip. (**a**) Supine radiograph of the pelvis. (**b**) Diagrammatic evaluation of the neonatal hip. N, ossification nucleus of the femoral head; AR, acetabular roof; T, triradiate cartilage. The left hip is normal. The right femoral head ossification nucleus is not in the lower inner quadrant, there is proximal migration of the femoral shaft, disruption of Shenton's curved line and the acetabular index is shallow. This is consistent with developmental dysplasia of the right hip

index is determined by drawing a straight line beginning at Hilgenreiner's line as it passes through the triradiate cartilage and continuing along the acetabular roof. The acetabular angle is the angle between Hilgenreiner's line and the line drawn along the acetabular roof. This angle should be less than 30°. The average normal angle is 27.5°. Values greater than 30° are consistent with DDH. The final measurement to be made is the distance between the femoral head or femoral metaphysis and Hilgenreiner's line. The distance is smaller on the abnormal side due to proximal migration of the femur.

Radiographic signs of DDH include small, asymmetrical femoral heads, delayed ossification of the femoral head, an acetabular roof angle greater than 30°, discontinuity in Shenton's line, and the formation of a neoacetabulum, lateralization or proximal migration of the femoral head[6]. The radiographic manifestation of DDH may not be present until the child is four to six months of age.

## Sonography

Sonography is able to image structures in the hip that are not identified on conventional radiographs during the neonatal period such as the cartilaginous femoral head, cartilaginous acetabular rim, and labrum (Figure 2). The size, shape, and position of the femoral head can be assessed sonographically before they are visualized radiographically. The motion of the femoral head in the acetabulum under stress can also be tested. Additionally, the shape of the acetabulum can be evaluated. Sonography is able to evaluate the morphologic development of the cartilaginous and bony acetabulum, labrum, femoral head, the degree to which the femoral head is covered by the labrum, the position of the femoral head in the

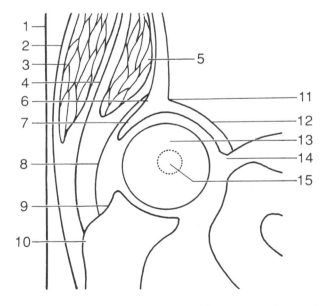

**Figure 2** Normal hip sonographic anatomy (coronal plane, neutral position). 1, skin; 2, subcutaneous fat; 3, gluteus medius muscle; 4, intermuscular septum; 5, gluteus minimis muscle; 6, acetabular cartilaginous rim; 7, acetabular limbus; 8, articular capsule; 9, osseo-cartilaginous border of femoral neck; 10, greater trochanter; 11, osseous acetabulum; 12, acetabular roof (ilium); 13, cartilaginous femoral head; 14, triradiate cartilage; 15, ossification nucleus of the femoral head

acetabulum at rest, during motion and stress. Indications for neonatal hip sonography include the presence of risk factors for developmental displacement of the hip, an abnormal hip examination, and the need to evaluate the response to treatment.

Sonography can typically be performed until the femoral head ossifies. Ossification of the femoral head begins between two and eight months of age, occurs earlier in girls than boys, and is often complete by one year. Once the femoral head is completely ossified, it is difficult to obtain adequate sonographic images due to artifact.

Real-time sonography is performed with a linear-array transducer. For patients up to the age of three months, a 7.5 MHz transducer is ideal; three to seven months, 5.0 MHz and after seven months, 3.0 MHz.

Sonographically, the femoral head is hypoechoic since it is cartilaginous and contains a focal echogenic ossification nucleus. The femoral head sits within the acetabulum which is echogenic and has a deep concave configuration. Two-thirds of the head should be covered by the labrum. The labrum is narrow and has a triangular shape. The labrum is composed of hyaline cartilage and is hypoechoic except at its tip which is echogenic due to its fibrous content. The femoral head should be stable within the acetabulum with stress after four weeks of age. During the neonatal period (i.e., the first four weeks of life) there is 'physiologic laxity' of the ligaments about the hip which allows the hip to be unstable[15].

There are two sonographic techniques used in the diagnosis of DDH: static (morphologic) and dynamic[16,17]. Although the dynamic approach is more commonly used and preferred, the techniques are not mutually exclusive. Results from both procedures can be integrated.

The static or morphologic technique was introduced in 1980 by Graf, an Austrian orthopedic surgeon[16]. The standard sonographic image is acquired in the coronal plane at the midacetabular level. This image includes the femoral head, acetabulum, labrum, and the iliac bone as it meets the triradiate cartilage. This produces a coronal image of the hip which has a configuration of an inverted 'Y' (Figure 3).

Graf utilized a series of lines and angle measurements to evaluate the morphology of the acetabulum[16,18] (Figure 4):

(1) The baseline connects the osseous acetabular convexity to the point where the joint capsule and pericondrium unite.

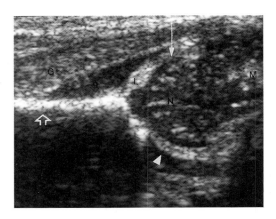

**Figure 3** Coronal – neutral sonogram of the hip at the midacetabular level. Open arrow, iliac wing; arrowhead, osseous acetabulum; arrow, cartilaginous acetabulum; m, femoral metaphysis; G, gluteus medius; g, gluteus minimus; L, labrum; N, ossification nucleus of the femoral head

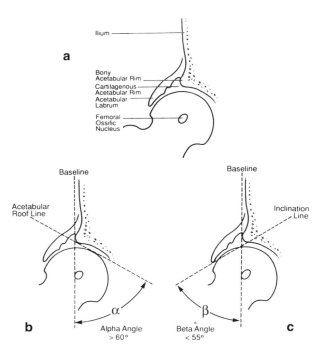

**Figure 4** Morphologic sonographic evaluation of the hip. (**a**) anatomic landmarks; (**b**) alpha angle; (**c**) beta angle

(2) The inclination line connects the osseous acetabular convexity to the labrum.

(3) The acetabular roof line connects the lower edge of the medially acetabular roof to the osseous acetabular convexity.

Based on the above lines, the alpha and beta angles are measured. The alpha angle is the angle between the baseline and the acetabular roof line and represents the osseous acetabulum. The alpha angle is normally > 60°. The beta angle is the angle between the baseline and the inclination line. This angle evaluates the formation and size of the cartilaginous acetabulum and is normally < 55°. The alpha angle reflects changes in the osseous portion of the acetabulum, which occur gradually. The beta angle reflects changes in the cartilaginous acetabulum, which occur more quickly than do changes in the osseous acetabulum and may therefore be more sensitive than the alpha angle[19].

According to the Graf classification there are four types of neonatal hips. The neonatal hip is classified according to its alpha and beta angles. A normal hip has an alpha angle of less than 60° and is classified as a type I hip. A type II hip has an alpha angle of between 43° and 60°. A type III hip has an alpha angle of less than 43° and a beta angle greater than 77°. In a type IV hip the alpha angle is less than 43° and the beta angle is immeasurable. Type I hips are normal and require no further evaluation. Type II hips must be monitored. Follow-up studies may be required. Type III and IV hips must be treated. Sonographic signs of developmental displacement of the hip include a shallow (dysplastic) acetabulum, delayed ossification of the femoral head, an inverted labrum, displacement of the femoral head (in either a lateral or posterior direction), increased thickness of the acetabular cartilage, an alpha angle > 60° and a beta angle < 55°. Although the sensitivity and specificity of sonography approaches 100%, a 'normal' sonogram does not absolutely exclude DDH.

Harcke and Graf formulated basic standards (Table 2) for dynamic hip sonography[20]. The hip is imaged in orthogonal planes: coronal (longitudinal) and transverse (axial) (Figure 5). Images of the hip (Figure 6) are obtained in coronal–extension, coronal–flexion, transverse–extension and transverse–flexion positions.

The examination begins with a coronal–neutral (Figure 3) or coronal–flexion image (Figure 6a). For the coronal–neutral image, the hip is held in 15–20° of flexion. This is considered physiological. For the coronal–flexion image, the hip is held in 90° of flexion. The images in the standard or midacetabular plane include the iliac bone as it meets the triradiate cartilage which should be in the middle of the field. The tip of the labrum must be included in this image. The sonographic images differ in that the echogenic femoral metaphysis is seen in the coronal–neutral position but not the coronal–flexion position. Both images are obtained with the transducer held in the coronal

**Table 2**  Sonography of the hip: dynamic standard minimum examination[17]

*Principles*

1.  The hip should be examined at rest and when stressed.
2.  Assessment should include views in orthogonal planes.
3.  Assessment includes description of both stability and morphology.

*Methods*

1.  Examination is performed with a real-time linear-array transducer.
2.  The examination may be done with the infant in a supine or lateral position.

*Components*

1.  Either A or B
    A.  Coronal–neutral view in standard planes at rest. Additional stress view optional. Validation by line/angle measurement optional.
    B.  Coronal–flexion view in standard plane at rest. Additional stress view optional. Validation by line/angle measurement optional.
2.  Transverse–flexion view with stress.

*Definition of terms*

1.  Coronal–neutral view: the transducer is oriented in a coronal plane with respect to the acetabulum. The hip is maintained in physiological neutral (slight flexion).
2.  Standard plane: a mid-acetabular plane is defined by a straight iliac line and the lip of the os ilium. The tip of the labrum must be identifiable in this plane.
3.  Stress: a telescopic or piston maneuver of the adducted hip, in a posterior direction to provoke dislocation. A reverse (stress) maneuver may be used to assess reduction.
4.  Transverse–flexion view: the transducer is oriented in a transverse (axial) plane with respect to the acetabulum (orthogonal to the coronal plane). The hip is in 90° of flexion.
5.  Coronal–flexion view: the transducer is oriented in a coronal plane with respect to the acetabulum. The hip is in 90° of flexion.

axis of the hip. In both cases, the femoral head should rest against the osseous acetabulum. Approximately two-thirds of the femoral head should be covered by the labrum. Stress can be applied in the coronal–flexion position by pistoning the hip. This is accomplished by pushing and pulling the hip in an anterior and posterior direction. If the hip is unstable, the femoral head

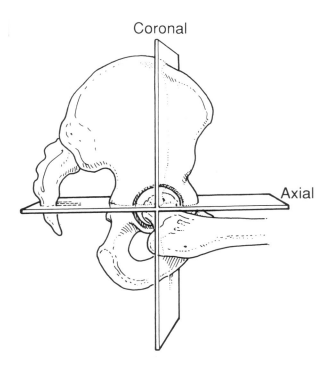

**Figure 5** Coronal and axial planes of the hip

will be identified posterior to the acetabulum. A coronal–extension image may also be obtained (Figure 6b).

The next step is the transverse–flexion image (Figure 6c). In this position, the transducer is held in the axial plane and the hip is held in 90° of flexion. The hip is pushed posteriorly and adducted in an attempt to dislocate the hip. This is analogous to the Barlow maneuver. If the hip dislocates, the examiner should be able to feel the femoral head dislocate. The hip is then pulled and abducted to attempt to reduce a dislocatable hip. This is analogous to the Ortolani maneuver. A transverse–extension can also be obtained (Figure 6d).

If the femoral head dislocates laterally, the center of the femoral head does not line up with the iliac wing (Figure 7). A line drawn through the

iliac wing will pass through the medial aspect of the femoral head. If the femoral head dislocates posteriorly, only an echogenic arc which represents one side of the femoral head is seen (Figure 8).

Stress view can be obtained with a 'piston maneuver'. The hip is placed in 90° of flexion and pressure is applied in the anterior and posterior direction. The transducer is held in the axial plane along the posterior and lateral aspect of the hip.

Hips are classified according to their behavior under stress as either normal, unstable, or dislocated (Table 3). The normal neonatal femoral head cannot be displaced out of the acetabulum but can have up to 6 mm of motion on the left and 4 mm of motion on the right during abduction and adduction due to physiological laxity. Unstable hips are further divided into subluxable and dislocatable. A subluxable hip is one in which the proximal femur moves (more than 6 mm on the left and 4 mm on the right) within the acetabulum but cannot be displaced out of it. A dislocatable hip is one in which the proximal femur can be displaced out of the acetabulum but can be reduced. A dislocated hip is one in which the femoral head is displaced out of the acetabulum and cannot be reduced.

## Treatment

The initial treatment of uncomplicated DDH is closed reduction. This may be accomplished by either placing two diapers on the neonate, or by the use of a spica cast, Pavlik harness, or brace. The hip should be positioned in flexion, with abduction and external rotation.

The position of the femoral head relative to the acetabulum can be determined with sonography, CT, and MRI. Sonography is preferred since it does not involve ionizing radiation. If sonography is performed on a patient with a cast, a 'window' must be cut into the case so that the transducer can be placed directly on the skin. Evaluation of the position of the femoral head with CT requires

**Table 3** Dynamic sonography classification[2]

| View and maneuver | Normal | Laxity with stress | Subluxed | Dislocatable/dislocated |
|---|---|---|---|---|
| Coronal–neutral (standard plane) | N | N | A | A |
| Coronal–flexion (standard plane) | N | N | A | A |
| Coronal–flexion (posterior lip) | N | N → A | A | A |
| No stress → piston stress | | | | |
| Transverse–flexion | | | | |
| abduction → adduction | N | N → A | N → A | A |

N, normal; A, abnormal

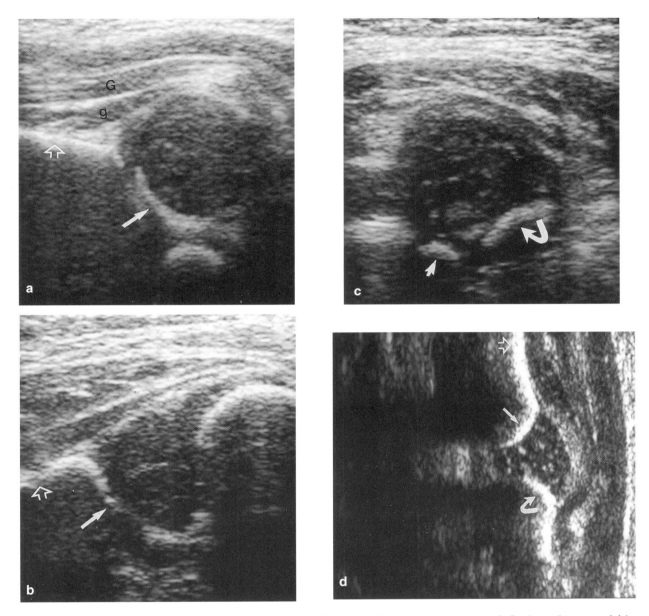

**Figure 6**   Dynamic sonographic evaluation of the hip. (**a**) normal hip sonogram, coronal–flexion; (**b**) normal hip sonogram, coronal–extension; (**c**) normal hip sonogram, transverse–flexion; (**d**) normal hip sonogram, transverse–extension. Arrow, pubic bone; curved arrow, ischium; long arrow, osseous acetabulum; I, ilium; L, labrum; G, gluteus medius; g, gluteus minimus

3 mm axial images through the hip. Evaluation with MRI requires 3 mm axial T1-weighted images. Intravenous contrast is not needed.

Causes of failure of closed reduction include inversion of the labrum or capsule and invagination of the iliopsoas muscle which can be imaged most efficiently by sonography and MRI. If closed reduction fails or if the dislocation is teratogenic the patient usually requires open reduction.

## Screening

Development of both sides of the neonatal hip (the acetabulum and femoral head) requires the femoral head to be seated normally within the acetabulum. If the femoral head and acetabulum are not in their normal position both sides of the hip will develop abnormally. This will cause abnormal morphology and function. If the

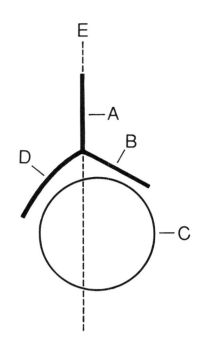

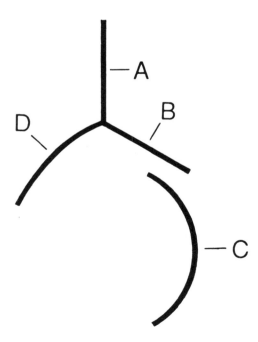

**Figure 7** Lateral dislocation of the hip. (**a**) sonogram; (**b**) diagram. The center of the femoral head does not line up with the center of the iliac wing (E). More than 50% of the femoral head is uncovered (lateral to the center of the iliac wing). This is consistent with a lateral dislocation. A, ileum; B, cartilaginous acetabulum; C, femoral head; D, acetabular medial roof

diagnosis is made early and treatment is instituted promptly a potentially abnormal hip may develop normally. The most important factor influencing outcome is the age at which the diagnosis is made and treatment initiated[1]. Treatment should begin before the patient walks. Sonography has been found to be more sensitive than physical examination in the detection of DDH[3,4]. The goal of screening sonography of the neonatal hip is to establish an early diagnosis so that treatment can be instituted as early as possible[21]. The ideal screening program will reduce the number of cases diagnosed late, i.e. after the neonatal period.

There is no uniform agreement on a neonatal sonographic screening strategy for DDH. Newborn screening programs are more developed in some parts of Europe than they are in the United States. The results of screening studies have been mixed. Some studies have found that routinely screening every newborn regardless of their risk factors or physical examination detects more positive cases than does physical examination alone[3,4,22]. Consequently, routine screening of all newborns seems advantageous. However, other studies have found that routine newborn screening did not reduce the number of cases which were diagnosed late[23]. Routine newborn screening is expensive and may lead to over-treatment since

**Figure 8** Posterior dislocation of the hip. Only an echogenic arc representing the femoral head is seen when the hip is flexed and adducted. This represents a posterior dislocation. A, ileum; B, cartilaginous acetabulum; C, femoral head; D, acetabular medial roof

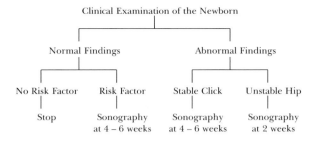

**Figure 9** Recommended screening algorithm for developmental displacement of the hip[2]

many cases of minor instability which will resolve without treatment will be detected. Newborn screening will not detect those cases which develop later in childhood. Therefore, universal screening sonography of every newborn hip has not been adopted in the United States.

Neonatal screening hip sonography is performed in the United States if the physical examination is abnormal, or if risk factors or associated congenital anomalies are present[2] (Figure 9). Harcke recommends that the hips of every patient who presents to the physician should be physically examined throughout childhood[16,20]. Patients who have a normal examination and no risk factors need no further work-up. If a hip is unstable, a screening sonogram should be performed at two weeks of age. Those that have a 'click' or a risk factor should have a screening sonogram at four to six weeks of age. This algorithm has been criticized because it does not diagnose those cases of developmental displacement of the hip that present late (i.e. beyond the neonatal period). However, the incidence of late presentation is low and will be diagnosed if every child has their hip physically examined during their visits to their physician[24]. Those patients who develop an abnormal physical examination should have either a hip sonogram or a pelvic radiograph depending on their age and the degree of ossification of the femoral head.

# References

1. Townstend DJ, Tolo V. Congenital dislocation of the hip. *Curr Opin Rheumatol* 1994;6:183–6
2. Harcke HT, Grissom LE. Infant hip sonography: current concepts. *Semin Ultrasound, CT, MRI* 1994;15:256–63
3. Rosendahl K, Markestad T, Lie RT. Congenital dislocation of the hip: a prospective study comparing ultrasound and clinical examination. *Acta Pediatr* 1992;81:177–81
4. Tonnis D, Storch K, Ulbrich H. Results of newborn screening for congenital dislocation of the hip with and without sonography and correlation of risk factors. *J Pediatr Orthop* 1990;10:142–52
5. Special Report. Screening for the detection of congenital dysplasia of the hip. *Archiv Dis Child* 1986;61:921–6
6. Dahnert W. *Radiology Review Manual*. Baltimore, MD: Williams and Wilkins, 1993:35–7
7. Hinderaker T, Daltveit AK, Irgens LM, *et al.* The impact of intra-uterine factors on neonatal hip instability. *Acta Orthop Scand* 1994;65:239–42
8. Amato M, Claus R, Huppi P. Perinatal hip assessment in very low birth weight infants. *Pediatr Radiol* 1992;22:361–2
9. Boal DKB, Schwentker EP. assessment of congenital hip dislocation with real-time ultrasound: a pictorial essay. *Clin Imag* 1991;15:77–90
10. Torisu T, Fujikawa Y, Yano H, *et al.* Association of HLA-DR and HLD-DQ antigens with congenital dislocation and dysplastic osteoarthritis of the hip in Japanese people. *Arthr Rheumat* 1993;36:815–18
11. Oski FA. *Principles and Practice of Pediatrics*. Philadelphia: JB Lippincott Company, 1994: 1018–20
12. Stanton RP, Capecci R. CT for early evaluation of developmental dysplasia of the hip. *J Pediatr Orthop* 1992;12:727–30
13. Atar D, Lehman WB, Grant AD. 2D and 3D CT and MRI in developmental dysplasia of the hip. *Orthop Rev* 1992;21:1189–97
14. Johnson ND, Wood BP, Jackman KV. Complex infantile and congenital hip dislocation: assessment with magnetic resonance imaging. *Radiology* 1988; 168:151–6
15. Keller MS, Weltin GG, Rattner Z, *et al.* Normal instability of the hip in the neonate: US standards. *Radiology* 1988;169:733–6
16. Graf R. The diagnosis of congenital hip joint dislocation by the ultrasonic compound treatment. *Archiv Orthop Traumat Surg* 1980;97:117–33
17. Harcke HT, Grissom LE. Performing dynamic sonography of the infant hip. *Am J Roentgenol* 1990;155:837–44
18. Graf R. Fundamentals of sonographic diagnosis of infant hip dysplasia. *J Pediatr Orthop* 1984;4: 735–40

19. Malkawi H, Asir B, Tadros F, *et al.* Sonographic image of the newborn hip with positive Ortolani's sign. *Clin Orthop Relat Res* 1992;279:138–43

20. Langer R. Ultrasonic investigation of the hip in newborns in the diagnosis of congenital hip dislocation: classification and results of a screening program. *Skelet Radiol* 1987;16:275–9

21. Harcke HT. Screening newborns for developmental displacement of the hip: the role of sonography. *Am J Roentgenol* 1994;152:395–7

22. Marks DS, Clegg J, Al-Chalabi AN. Routine ultrasound screening for neonatal hip instability: can we abolish late-presentation congenital dislocation of the hip? *J Bone Joint Surg* (Br Vol) 1994;76B:534–8

23. Clarke NMP, Clegg J, Al-Chalabi AN. Ultrasound screening of hips at risk for congenital hip dysplasia: failure to reduce the incidence of late cases. *J Bone Joint Surg* 1989;71B:9–12

24. Hazel JR, Beals RK. Diagnosing dislocation of the hip in infancy. *West J Med* 1989;151:39–41

# Sonography of the neonatal spinal canal

11

*Michael A. DiPietro and Kimberly A. Garver*

The spinal canal and its contents can be demonstrated sonographically with great clarity in the neonatal period. The suspected occult tethered spinal cord, various dysraphic conditions, and the relationship of back masses and midline cutaneous deformities to the spinal canal are among the indications for spine sonography. Sonography can be performed easily and at the bedside. Sonographic findings have concurred with those on magnetic resonance imaging (MRI) in a recent comparative study of both modalities in children[1]. Visualization in the neonatal period is especially clear and compares favorably with MRI. The availability of high resolution high frequency transducers from many ultrasound vendors now leaves operator inexperience as the main reason for unsuccessful neonatal spinal sonography. We hope that this chapter will not only show the anatomy and pathology which can be displayed sonographically, but that it will give the reader sufficient clinical background and information on technique to be able to try spinal sonography.

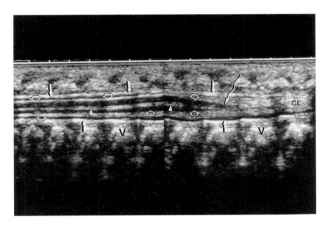

**Figure 1** Composite longitudinal sonogram of the low thoracic to mid-lumbar spinal canal (patient's head is to the left). The caudal end of the spinal cord (open arrowheads) widens above the tapered conus medullaris (wavy arrow). The central echo complex in the center of the cord appears as two parallel lines (small arrowheads). Straight arrows, dura; V, vertebral body (only two are labelled); CE, cauda equina

## Technique

Incomplete ossification of the posterior spinal elements allows sonography to provide a broad panoramic view of the neonatal spinal canal and its contents (Figure 1). A posterior approach is used with the patient prone or lateral decubitus, but the examination could be performed with the baby being held upright or sitting[2,3]. It is crucial that the spine be flexed enough to separate the posterior spinal elements. When prone, this is accomplished by having the baby lie over a small pillow or a rolled sheet. Slight elevation of the upper part of the body will better distend the caudal aspect of the thecal sac[4]. Care must be taken that flexion is not so extreme as to compromise the infant's breathing. This consideration is amplified if the baby has been sedated. However, in our experience sedation in the neonatal period has never been necessary. If the baby is not hungry, he or she will often fall asleep during the scanning. The gentle rubbing of the back by the transducer and warm coupling gel is apparently soothing to most infants.

Seven-MHz transducers generally work well in neonates. Higher frequencies (10–12 MHz) also work in some. A 5-MHz transducer might be needed if the baby is unusually large, and is used in older infants. Our personal preference is for linear array transducers, but curved array or sector transducers can be used. We employ the latter in special situations where the body surface is curved such as at the cranio-cervical junction or at the margin of a meningocele. Scanning is performed in midline sagittal (longitudinal) and axial (transverse) planes, the latter mainly between spinous processes. It is not usually necessary to obtain sagittal images off midline, at an angle and between lamina, as it is in older children who have more completely ossified posterior elements. Sagittal images are usually oriented with the baby's head toward the left on the viewing screen, similar to conventional abdominal images. However, on transverse scans we usually have the patient's right on the viewer's right, which is the opposite of common practice in the rest of the body. Our reason for this is that with the baby lying prone our orientation matches the body as viewed from the feet, and scanning movements of the transducer on the patient's back will correspond in direction to those on the viewing screen. We have found this orientation helpful in cases with complex and asymmetric anatomy and pathology.

Since most examinations are performed to exclude an occult tethered spinal cord, determining the vertebral level of the tip of the conus medullaris is most important and, accordingly, the lumbar spinal canal receives the most attention. However, the entire canal can be examined, and in the neonate we usually study the spinal canal at all levels. The transducer's depth of field is adjusted so that the vertebral bodies are at the bottom of the image. The spinal canal is usually easily identified and the depth of the image field adjusted accordingly. When first learning spinal sonography it helps to scan the sacral region first, where the canal is easily identified by the stepwise ascent of the sacral vertebral elements, and follow the spinal canal craniad (Figure 2). A stand-off pad is helpful to examine the soft tissues dorsal to the spine, such as looking for a sinus tract. This area is also best studied with high frequency near-field transducers, such as those which have been developed for musculoskeletal and small parts sonography. Oscillations of the spinal cord and roots of the cauda equina are observed best when the image persistence or frame averaging is minimized.

## Normal anatomy

An understanding of pathological conditions requires first an appreciation of normal anatomy. Both are well demonstrated by sonography in the neonate[2,3,5–9] (Figure 1). The spinal canal is defined anteriorly by the echogenic posterior vertebral body surfaces and posteriorly by the posterior dorsal spinal elements, some of which might be incompletely ossified. The dura is visible as an echogenic line just internal to these osseous borders. The spinous processes appear as inverted 'U's. Lamina are seen when scanning slightly off midline and appear similar to overlapping roof tiles (Figure 3). The coccyx is mostly or completely unossified and therefore hypoechoic[10] (Figure 4). The spinal cord is hypoechoic with slightly echogenic borders and an echogenic line extending longitudinally along its midline. This

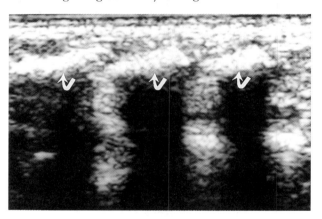

**Figure 3** Detailed off midline longitudinal view which shows lamina (curved arrows) resembling overlapping roof tiles

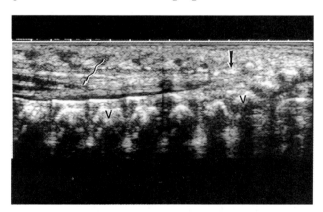

**Figure 2** Composite longitudinal sonogram of the lumbo-sacral spinal canal showing the conus tip (wavy arrow) and echogenic roots of the cauda equina. Patient's head is to the left. Straight arrow, caudal end of the thecal sac; V, vertebral body (only two are labelled)

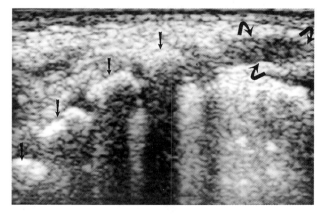

**Figure 4** Longitudinal view of the normal neonatal sacrum showing the 'stepwise' dorsal progression of the ossified sacral vertebral body segments (straight arrows) and the unossified coccyx (curved arrows)

central echo complex represents or is close to the cord's central canal[11,12] (Figure 1). A sonographic study of a coronally bisected cord specimen made a compelling case for the central echo complex being the dorsal extent of the cord's ventral median fissure[13]. The size and shape of the spinal cord vary along its length[5,9,14,15] (Figure 5). Its diameter is narrowest in the mid-thoracic levels and widest at the cervico-thoracic and thoraco-lumbar junctions. Transverse dentate ligaments of the cord are sometimes visible (Figure 6). The cord tapers caudally at the conus medullaris (Figure 5e). The nerve roots which surround the spinal cord are echogenic. They are especially noticeable

at and below the conus forming the cauda equina. Dorsal and ventral nerve roots can have a spider-like configuration at the tip of the conus in the transverse view (Figure 7). Clusters of normal nerve roots might be mistaken for an echogenic intracanalicular mass. Nerves, however, will be observed to move and change configuration as one scans along the canal in real-time. In transverse views nerve roots might appear as an echogenic clump in the middle of the spinal canal or as bilateral clusters (Figures 8 and 9), sometimes in an upside down 'V' configuration (Figure 10). Another potential false-positive finding is the bilateral dorsal and ventral roots at the very tip of

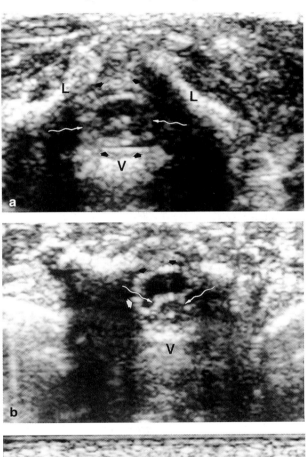

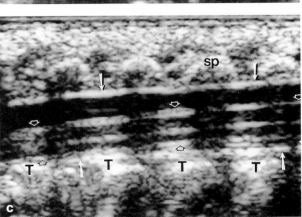

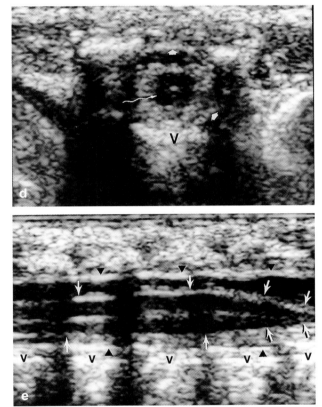

**Figure 5 (a–e)**   The normal spinal cord at various levels. Note the central echo complex in the middle of the cord appearing as a line in the longitudinal views and as a dot in the transverse views. L, lamina; V, vertebral body; T, thoracic vertebral body; sp, spinous process; small arrowheads, dura. (**a**) Transverse cervical cord (high-lighted by wavy arrows). (**b**) Transverse thoracic cord (highlighted by wavy arrows). Note how it is in the ventral aspect of the canal and smaller in diameter than the cervical or lumbar cord. (**c**) Longitudinal thoracic cord (highlighted by open arrowheads). The dura (arrows in this example) appears as thick echogenic bands along the canal. (**d**) Transverse lumbar cord (wavy arrow). (**e**) Longitudinal low thoracic-lumbar cord (highlighted by arrows). Note the tapered conus medullaris

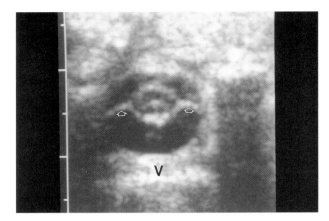

**Figure 6** Transverse view showing dentate ligaments (arrowheads) extending from the thoracic cord. V, vertebral body

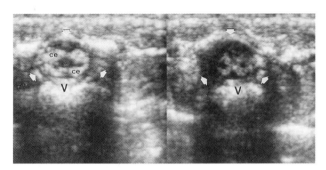

**Figure 7** Transverse views at the level of the conus on a split screen. The left frame shows the conus surrounded by echogenic dorsal and ventral roots of the cauda equina (ce). At the very tip of the conus (right frame) the dorsal and ventral roots have a 'spiderlike' or 'wavy X' configuration. V, vertebral body; arrowheads, dura

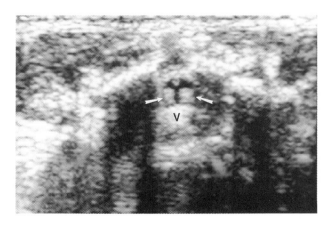

**Figure 8** Transverse view of the low lumbar canal showing cauda equina as bilateral clusters of nerve roots (arrows). V, vertebral body

the conus which can superficially mimic a split cord, diastematomyelia (vide infra) (Figures 11

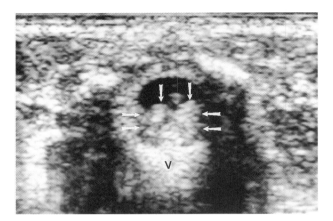

**Figure 9** Transverse view of the low lumbar canal in another infant showing cauda equina as bilateral clusters of nerve roots (arrows). V, vertebral body

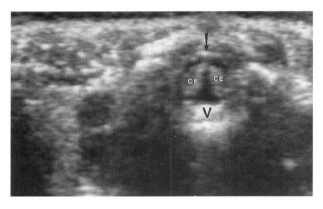

**Figure 10** Transverse view of the low lumbar canal showing cauda equina (ce) as bilateral clusters of nerve roots in an inverted 'V' configuration. Arrow, dorsal dura; V, vertebral body

and 12). Although they appear similar on the static image, they are readily distinguished during real-time scanning in both projections, above and below the area of concern.

The spinal cord and roots of the cauda equina are normally observed to move[16]. This is best seen with minimal frame persistence. Dorso-ventral oscillations occur at the frequency of the heartbeat, and there is also a superimposed motion which occurs with respirations. These movements are variably present in neonates but are almost always seen after one or two months of age.

## Level of the conus medullaris

The single most important determination is usually the level of the tip of the tapered conus medullaris. The normal level is in the upper lumbar canal, above the superior endplate of L3, with most cords ending above L2[17]. Normal levels are the same throughout infancy and childhood as determined by a cross-sectional study of normal children[18]. Another study concentrated exclusively on neonates and found that conus levels tend to be in the low normal range in premature newborns[19].

One has a general idea of the lumbar vertebral level by simply looking at the baby's back during the scanning examination. A transverse projection across the midline from the lowest palpable rib end is often L2[18]. A similar projection from the palpated apex of the iliac crest is often L5[18]. One can count vertebral levels on ultrasound by counting caudad from the lowest rib-bearing

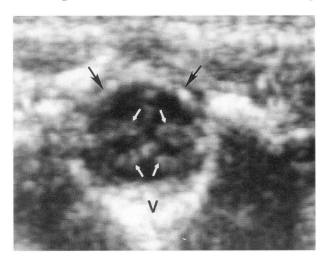

**Figure 11**  Transverse view of the tip of the conus medullaris. Dorsal and ventral nerve roots (white arrows) have a 'spiderlike' or 'wavy X' configuration. Note the vague 'similarity' to Figure 12. Black arrows, dorsal dura; V, vertebral body

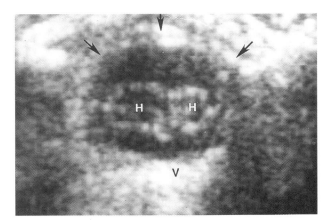

**Figure 12**  Transverse view of diastematomyelia. The septum traversing the spinal cord is not visible at this level, although the two hemicords (H) are clearly shown. Arrows, dorsal dura; V, vertebral body

vertebra or by counting craniad from the caudal end of the thecal sac (usually S2[20]), from the coccyx, or from the lumbosacral junction (Figure 13). The latter is identified as it is on lateral spine radiographs, by the angle formed by the lines projected along the posterior aspects of the lumbar and the sacral vertebral bodies[21]. One can also sonographically identify the lowest rib over each kidney and follow it medially to its vertebral body[18] (Figure 14). That level can be assigned as T12, although it could be off by a level if the patient has 11 or 13 pairs of ribs. If the conus tip is mid-lumbar, its exact level might therefore need to be determined by a correlative radiograph. The conus tip is carefully noted in both longitudinal and transverse sonographic projections and this position is marked on the skin by a radiopaque marker, such as a nipple marker used in chest radiography. In our experience most tethered cords have been unquestionably low and correlative radiographs were not usually needed.

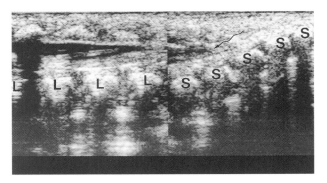

**Figure 13**  Longitudinal split screen composite view of the lumbosacral canal. The caudal end of the thecal sac (wavy arrow) usually corresponds to S2. L, lumbar vertebral bodies; S, sacral vertebral bodies

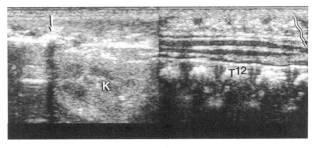

**Figure 14**  Longitudinal split screen showing a method of estimating the vertebral level of the conus tip (wavy arrow). Left frame identifies the lowest rib (straight arrow) over the kidney (K). In the right frame the rib is sonographically followed back to the vertebral column to presumably locate T12. Note the two minimally separated parallel lines extending longitudinally down the middle of the cord, the central echo complex

Sometimes the conus tip is obscured by an overlying posterior spinal element, but this is more often a problem in older infants and children. In those cases the conus level is inferred as lying between the lowest level showing cord and the adjacent caudal level which contains only cauda equina[18].

## Pathologic findings

Although spinal sonography is performed predominantly to study the contents of the spinal canal, osseous anomalies are sometimes demonstrated (Figure 15a,b). However, the most common and important request is to look for the occult tethered cord. The tethered spinal cord is 'a pathologic fixation of the spinal cord in an abnormal caudal location, so that the cord suffers mechanical stretching, distortion, and ischemia with daily activities, growth, and development'[22]. It is usually associated with a mass of the lower cord or filum terminale[23–25] (Figure 16). The mass, which often has lipomatous elements, can be continuous with the subcutaneous tissues and present as a fatty lump on the lower back (Figure 16f,g). Lipomas can be isolated to the filum terminale or extend to and infiltrate the spinal cord and conus medullaris to varying degrees[7,23,24,26] (Figure 16d,e,f,g). Lipomas can be small or large and are usually echogenic.

The tethered spinal cord, in addition to being in a more caudal location, is often fixed eccentrically within the canal (Figure 16c,d). Spinal cord oscillations might be diminished in the tethered cord. If cord oscillations are present distant from the site of tethering, they are often dampened or absent closer to the point of fixation[2,27,28]. However, since normal brisk oscillations of the cord are not as apparent in normal neonates as in older infants, looking for dampened or absent oscillations in neonates with tethered cords has limited usefulness (false positives). Most non-oscillating cords in neonates are normal and are not due to tethering. In addition, the tethered cord often oscillates freely in the young infant beyond the neonatal period (false negatives). However, the oscillations usually diminish as the child grows, presumably because the cord is anchored and is being stretched[22,29].

Hydromelia is another sonographically observable abnormality of the spinal cord which can be seen in variable degrees (Figures 17 and 18). One should first be aware that slight prominence of the central canal at the caudal end of the cord is a common finding in neonates[30–32]

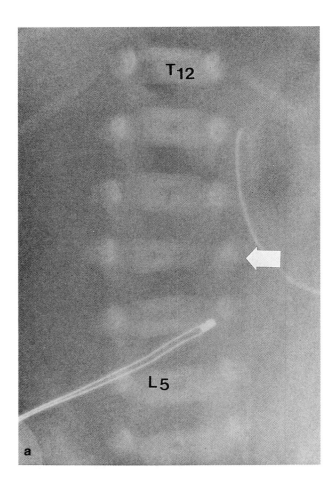

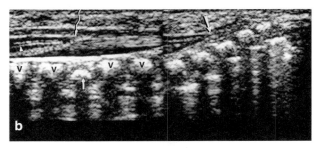

**Figure 15** (a) Hypoplastic vertebral body. Antero-posterior projection (AP) radiograph showing the hypoplastic left portion of L3 vertebral body (arrow). $T_{12}$, vertebral body 12th thorax; $L_5$, vertebral body 5th lumbar. (b) Hypoplastic vertebral body. Split screen composite longitudinal sonogram of the lumbosacral canal. The hypoplastic mid-lumbar vertebral body (small straight arrow) is noted in contrast to the other lumbar vertebral bodies (V). Incidental note is made of two minimally separated lines in the middle of the cord (small arrowhead) which constitute the central echo complex. Wavy arrow, tip of normal conus; large straight arrow, caudal tip of thecal sac

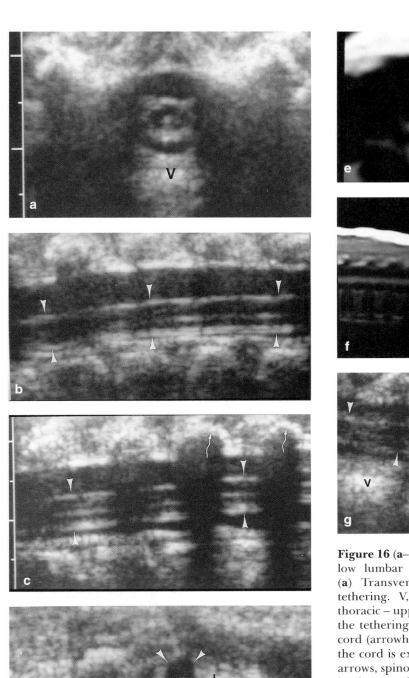

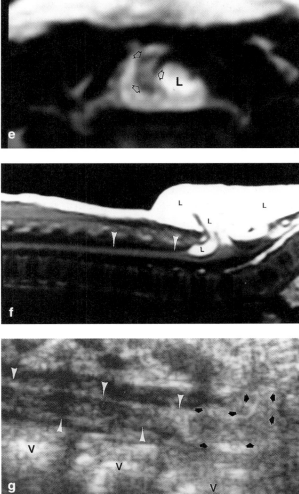

**Figure 16 (a–g)** Spinal cord tethered by a lipoma in the low lumbar canal shown on sonography and MRI. (**a**) Transverse mid-lumbar cord, cephalad to the tethering. V, vertebral body. (**b**) Longitudinal lower thoracic – upper lumbar cord (arrowheads) cephalad to the tethering. (**c**) Longitudinal view of the mid-lumbar cord (arrowheads), cephalad to the tethering. Note that the cord is extending dorsally as well as caudally. Wavy arrows, spinous processes. (**d**) Transverse view of the low lumbar canal showing the cord (arrowheads) tethered dorsally and caudally by an intracanalicular lipoma (L) on its right. (**e**) Transverse MRI of the low lumbar canal in same orientation as sonogram (i.e. dorsal is up) showing the cord (arrowheads) tethered dorsally and caudally by an intracanalicular lipoma (L) on its right. (**f**) Sagittal MRI of lumbosacral canal showing cord (arrowheads) tethered at the lumbosacral junction by a lipoma (L) which extends from the subcutaneous tissues to the spinal cord. (**g**) Sagittal sonogram of the cord (white arrowheads) tethered in the low lumbar canal by the lipoma (black arrowheads). V, vertebral bodies

(Figures 1, 14 and 15b). Focal hydromyelia is often present just cephalad to the site of tethering in dysraphic conditions as myelomeningocele or lipomyelomeningocele[33–35]. Hydromyelia might also accompany diastematomyelia, a condition in which the cord is split at one or more sites by an osseous, cartilaginous, or fibrous septum[36–38] (Figure 12). The two segments of the cord can be seen most clearly on transverse views. They might rejoin caudal to the cleft. The vertebral column is virtually always abnormal on plain radiography in patients with diastematomyelia[7].

Small 'cysts' in the filum terminale might be remnants of a terminal ventricle or an 'arachnoid pseudocyst' and of no significance[30,31]. Cysts can be detected sonographically. An example of a cyst in the cauda equina region was seen together with a thick filum terminale (Figure 19). In another case, a very thin walled cyst on the dorsal aspect of the low thoracic cord was discovered on sonography. It caused slight focal flattening of the dorsal surface of the underlying cord (Figure 20a), a finding which was corroborated on a subsequent MRI (Figure 20b,c) and at surgery.

The main reason for studying the cord in cases of clinically obvious myelomeningocele or myeloschisis is to exclude additional cord pathology such as diastematomyelia[6,39]. Dural and filar fibrolipomas and leptomyelolipomas can also occur with myelomeningocele[24]. The importance of detecting associated anomalies cephalad or caudal to the neural placode is that, if they are not recognized and repaired, they could lead to late symptomatic re-tethering of the spinal cord following closure of the myelomeningocele[40]. Experience with intraoperative sonography has provided a clear picture of pathologic anatomy[41]. This knowledge can be transferred to the pre-operative neonate with an open or covered dysraphic defect. The entire

spinal canal can be studied easily to the margin of the skin defect. In addition and if requested, the membrane-covered or open spine defect can be studied through a thin clear plastic drape which has been placed over it to prevent contamination. Care should be taken that no pressure be applied while scanning on the defect. The anatomy of the cord, adhesion of the cord to the dorsal aspect of the spinal canal cephalad to the defect, and the appearance of the neural placode and nerve roots in the defect can all be seen on sonography (Figure 21). Sonography of the defect *per se* is more often requested in ambiguous cases to distinguish a meningocele from a myelomeningocele or if the dysraphic defect is skin-covered. Myelomeningocele

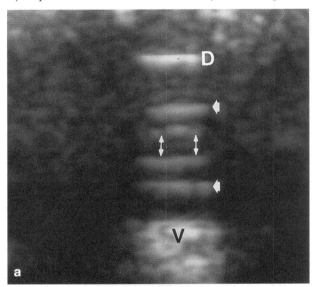

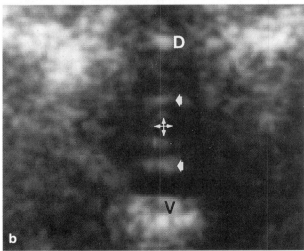

**Figure 18** Longitudinal (**a**) and transverse (**b**) segmental views (obtained between shadowing posterior elements) of a hydromyelic spinal cord. Arrowheads, dorsal and ventral cord margins; double headed arrows, hydromyelia; D, dorsal dura; V, vertebral body

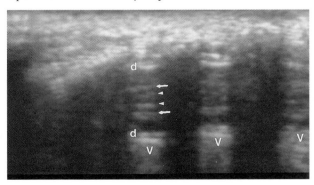

**Figure 17** A segmented longitudinal view showing hydromyelia as wide separation of the central echoes (arrowheads) in the central portion of the cord (arrows). d, dura; V, vertebral bodies

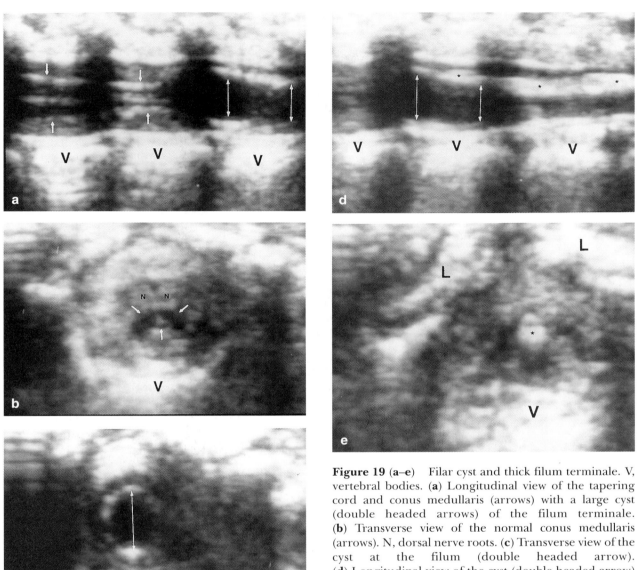

**Figure 19 (a–e)** Filar cyst and thick filum terminale. V, vertebral bodies. (a) Longitudinal view of the tapering cord and conus medullaris (arrows) with a large cyst (double headed arrows) of the filum terminale. (b) Transverse view of the normal conus medullaris (arrows). N, dorsal nerve roots. (c) Transverse view of the cyst at the filum (double headed arrow). (d) Longitudinal view of the cyst (double headed arrow) and the thick filum terminale (*). (e) Transverse view of the thick echogenic filum terminal (*). L, lamina

shows a flat non-tubulated cord (neural placode) with nerve roots extending into the defect[42]. The nerve roots drop from the neural placode with dorsal roots lateral and ventral roots medial. A meningocele, in contrast, often shows nothing but fluid within the sac (Figure 22). However, a meningocele can also contain fine lace-like strands extending into the sac (Figure 23). They are finer than nerve roots and are strands of lining tissue, such as arachnoid. Although the spinal cord is tubulated and does not enter the sac in a meningocele, the cord might be focally eccentric in the canal and even be tethered by a focal adhesion (Figure 23).

Virtually all children with a myelomeningocele also have a Chiari II (i.e. Arnold–Chiari) malformation. Obliteration of the cisterna magna between the cerebellum and occipital bone is apparent on standard cranial sonography (Figure 24). However, more detailed lower hindbrain and cervical manifestations of this malformation can be studied from a posterior cervical approach[8,43,44]. Transverse images can be performed with the linear array transducer as was used for the rest of the spinal canal. It can also be used for sagittal images, but a sector or curved face transducer is helpful for sagittal imaging at the occipito-cervical junction. The normal cranio-cervical junction and

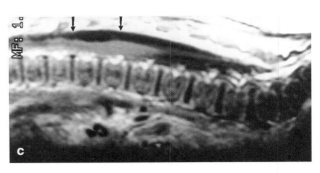

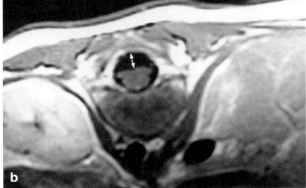

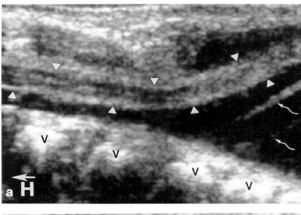

Figure 20 (a–c) Thin walled extramedullary cyst (arrows) on the dorsum of the low thoracic cord. Note how it slightly flattens the dorsal surface of the cord. (a) Sonogram; split screen (transverse view on left; longitudinal on right). (b) Transverse MRI. (c) Longitudinal MRI

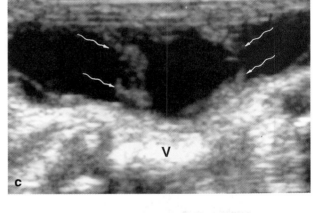

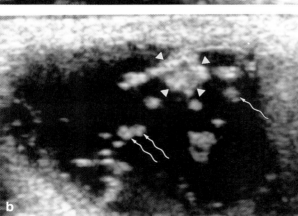

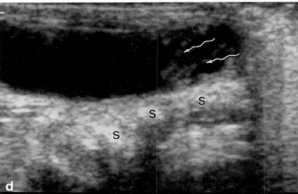

Figure 21 (a–d) Newborn with an unrepaired myelomeningocele. (a) and (b) Longitudinal (a) and transverse (b) views of lower cord (arrowheads) entering the dorsal sac. Note the increased echogenicity of the portion of the cord which extends into the sac. Wavy arrows, nerve roots (not all are labelled); V, vertebral bodies. H arrow points cephalad.(c) Transverse view of nerve roots (wavy arrows) extending ventrally from the neural placode in the dorsal, caudal aspect of the sac. V, vertebral body. (d) Longitudinal view of nerve roots (wavy arrows) extending ventrally and slightly cephalad from the dorsal, caudal aspect of the sac. S, sacral vertebral bodies

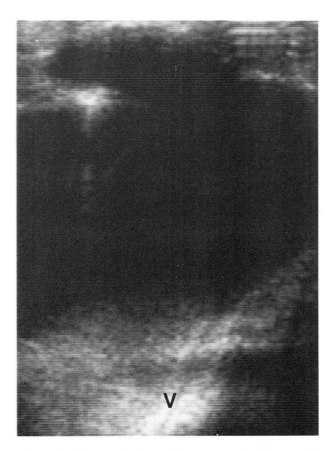

**Figure 22** Sagittal view of an unrepaired neonatal meningocele. Note how empty it is. V, vertebral body

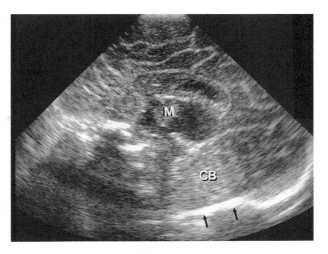

**Figure 24** Midline sagittal cranial sonogram obtained through the anterior fontanelle of a newborn with myelomeningocele and a Chiari II (i.e. Arnold-Chiari) malformation. The cerebellum (CB) is low, abutting the floor of the posterior fossa (arrows) and obliterating the cisterna magna. M, prominent interthalamic massa intermedia

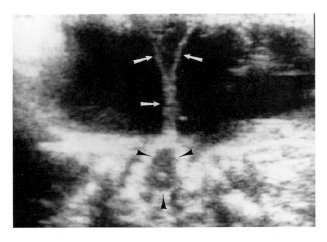

**Figure 23** Transverse view of the lumbar cord at the level of an unrepaired meningocele in a newborn. The spinal cord (black arrowheads) is within the spinal canal. In this case the shape of the cord is distorted dorsally by strands of lace-like pia-arachnoid (white arrow) which extend dorsally into the meningocele

cervical canal have anechoic cerebrospinal fluid (CSF) dorsal to the cervical spinal cord (Figure 25). In contrast, this dorsal anechoic space is diminished or absent in the Chiari II malformation since it is filled with ectopic herniated cerebellar vermis, the so-called vermian peg or vermian tongue (Figure 26). The medulla and 4th ventricle can also extend caudally into the cervical canal. Lower medulla can overlap and lie dorsal to upper cervical cord. This configuration is called the cervico-medullary kink (Figure 26a). The extent of vermian peg and the cervico-medullary kink can be seen on newborn cervical spine sonography. The anatomy is best appreciated from a comparison with MRI (Figure 27) or intra-operative sonography (Figure 28). We have not seen a dilated cervical 4th ventricle or a cervical extra-axial cyst or CSF loculation in a neonate as has been seen on intraoperative sonography in older children during Chiari II cervical decompression[45,46]. Perhaps these abnormalities develop over time. Since nearly all patients with myelomeningocele have a Chiari II malformation, merely confirming its presence is of little significance. Neurosurgeons might find it important to know the extent of malformation, and sonography can provide a quick assessment which can later be more thoroughly evaluated by MRI. Rarely is such detailed delineation required immediately in the newborn period.

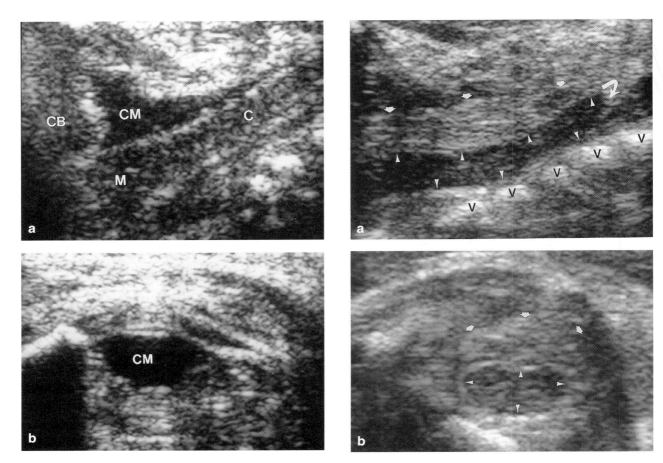

**Figure 25** Sagittal (**a**) and transverse (**b**) views of a normal upper cervical canal at the foramen magnum. CB, cerebellum; CM, cisterna magna; M, medulla; C, cervical cord

**Figure 26** Sagittal (**a**) and transverse (**b**) views of the cervical spinal canal in a patient with Chiari II malformation which were obtained through the intact skin and spine. Thick arrowheads, caudally displaced thick vermian peg; thin arrowheads, caudally displaced medulla and cervical cord; curved arrow, cervicomedullary kink; V, cervical vertebral bodies

## Other indications and associations

Midline cutaneous abnormalities over the lower back have been the most common reason for requesting neonatal spinal sonography. Midline dimples over the lower back occur in approximately 2–4.3% of newborns[47,48]. Most are low sacral or coccygeal pits without an associated tethered cord[32,49,50,51]. The superficial tissues are best studied with a high (7 or 10+ MHz) frequency transducer which has good near-field spatial resolution. The use of a stand-off pad between the skin and transducer face can also improve clarity of the superficial and subcutaneous tissue layers. A tract can sometimes be seen and followed, especially if it is fluid filled or if it disrupts normal soft tissue planes[49,52] (Figure 29). The soft tissue interfaces are continuous uninterrupted echogenic lines between skin, subcutaneous fat, muscle, and fascia. A sinus tract will disrupt the echogenic line and might be seen extending to the dura.

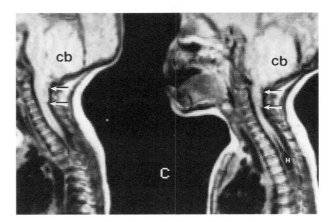

**Figure 27** Sagittal MRI of a Chiari II malformation. The vermian peg (arrows) extends through the foramen magnum into the upper cervical canal. cb, cerebellum; H, hydromyelia of the thoracic cord

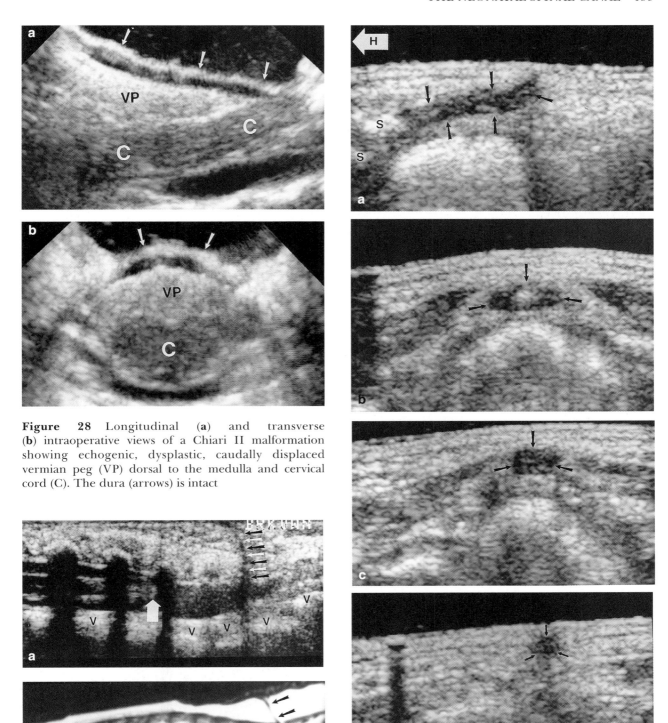

**Figure 28** Longitudinal (**a**) and transverse (**b**) intraoperative views of a Chiari II malformation showing echogenic, dysplastic, caudally displaced vermian peg (VP) dorsal to the medulla and cervical cord (C). The dura (arrows) is intact

**Figure 29** Sagittal sonogram (**a**) and MRI (**b**) showing a sinus tract (small arrows) dorsal to the sacral canal. Broad arrow, tip of the conus medullaris; V, vertebral bodies

**Figure 30** (**a–d**) Normal unossified coccyx (arrows) obtained through a stand-off pad. (**a**) Sagittal view of coccyx and ossified sacral elements (S). (**b**), (**c**) and (**d**) Transverse views of the coccyx in descending order. The most cephalad portion (**b**) includes the last sacral ossific nucleus. The most caudal portion (**d**) is right under the skin

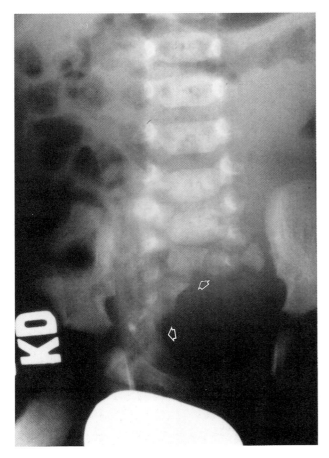

**Figure 31** Frontal radiograph of an infant with an anterior meningocele and a crescentic scimitar sacrum (arrowheads)

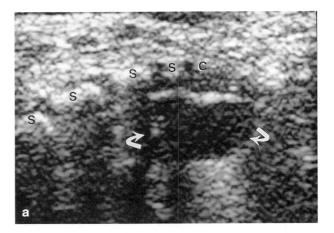

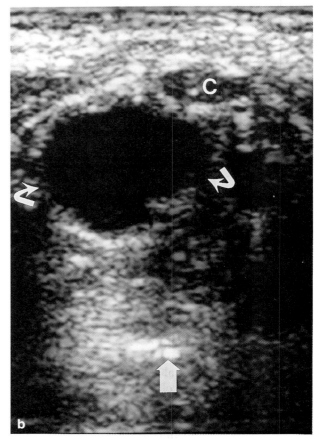

**Figure 32** Longitudinal (**a**) and transverse (**b**) views of a presacral cyst (curved arrows). S, sacral vertebral bodies; C, coccyx; broad arrow, air which had been instilled into the rectum for localization

However, dural penetration is difficult to ascertain or exclude on sonography[49]. We usually indicate in our report that 'although nothing abnormal was found and the spinal cord is not tethered, a hairline sinus tract cannot be entirely excluded'. The neonatal coccyx is usually of very low echogenicity and should not be mistaken for a cyst or fluid collection[10] (Figure 30).

During the first month of gestation the neural tube is closing while neural and epithelial tissues are differentiating from the overlying ectoderm. The concurrence of these events might explain the coincidence of midline cutaneous and spinal defects[50]. Midline hair patches, fatty lumps, skin tags, pigmented nevi, lumbar dimples, aplasia cutis, and hemangiomas over the back should prompt a search for an occult tethered spinal cord[49,50,53,54]. The exact percentage of children with these cutaneous abnormalities who have tethered cords is not known[47,50]. However, hemangiomas seem to have a high association with tethered spinal cord[53].

We routinely perform spinal sonography on neonates with imperforate anus, a malformation which has been associated with tethered cord[55-60]. Tethered cord has been seen in cases of high and low imperforate anus and in cases with minimal plain spinal radiographic findings[61].

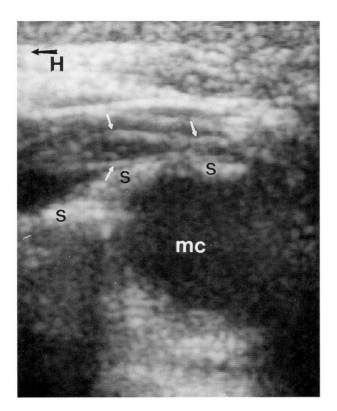

**Figure 33** Longitudinal view of the caudal aspect of the sacrum showing a low tethered spinal cord (arrows) and an anterior, pre-sacral meningocele (mc). S, sacral vertebral elements; H, cephalod direction

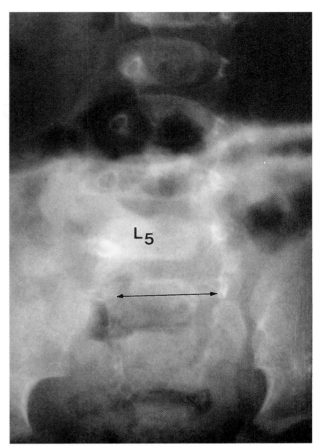

**Figure 34** Frontal radiograph shows widened interpediculate distance (arrow) in a patient with a posterior sacral myelomeningocele. A meningocele or a lipomyelomeningocele could have a similar appearance

A scimitar or crescentic sacrum occurs in 35% of patients with anorectal anomalies[60]. However, it also occurs without imperforate anus and warrants looking for a tethered cord (Figure 31). The anomalous sacrum can be appreciated on sonography, especially if it is asymmetric. The Currarino triad of scimitar sacrum, anal stenosis, and a pre-sacral dermoid or meningocele has been described[62,63]. The presacral mass can be visualized (Figure 32) and we have seen it associated with a tethered cord (Figure 33). A familial occurrence has been reported in some cases[62–64]. In an infant without an obvious open dysraphic spine, a wide interpediculate distance on the plain radiograph is suspicious for an occult spinal cord anomaly or tethering (Figure 34). However, one cannot rely on plain radiographs to entirely exclude dysraphism in a neonate[65]. Plain radiographs can appear normal, especially since the neonate's posterior spinal elements are often incompletely ossified.

Although a myelomeningocele will have a clinically determinable spinal level of neurologic dysfunction at birth (for example L3), an occult tethered cord, such as from a thick filum terminale or a lipoma, is often neurologically subtle or silent at birth. Problems with anal and urethral sphincter tone, postural foot deformities, and progressive scoliosis can develop as the child grows but are not usually manifest in the neonate. This correlates with the cord being tethered but not stretched until the child grows. We have seen cases where the asymptomatic infant has a low but freely oscillating cord which becomes less oscillating as the child grows and becomes symptomatic from the tethered cord. However, one must remember that in the neonatal period oscillations are often normally much more subtle than they are after one or two months of age.

In summary, sonography is an effective method which provides a quick and thorough look at the neonate's spinal canal with demonstration of normal and pathologic anatomy.

# References

1. Rohrschneider WK, Forsting M, Darge K, *et al*. Diagnostic value of spinal US: comparative study with MR in pediatric patients. *Radiology* 1996; 200:383–8

2. DiPietro MA, Venes JL. Real-time sonography of the pediatric spinal cord. Horizons and limits. *Concepts Pediatr Neurosurg* 1988;8:120–32

3. Zieger M, Dörr U. Pediatric spinal sonography. Part I: Anatomy and examination technique. *Pediatr Radiol* 1988;18:9–13

4. Naidich TP, Fernbach SK, McLone DG, *et al*. Sonography of the caudal spine and back: congenital anomalies in children. *Am J Radiol* 1984;142:1229–42

5. Gusnard DA, Naidich TP, Yousefzadeh DK, *et al*. Ultrasonic anatomy of the normal neonatal and infant spine: correlation with cryomicrotome sections and CT. *Neuroradiology* 1986;28:493–511

6. Jequier S, Cramer B, O'Gorman AM. Ultrasound of the spinal cord in neonates and infants. *Ann Radiol* 1985;28:225–31

7. Naidich TP, Radkowski MA, Britton J. Real-time sonographic display of caudal spinal anomalies. *Neuroradiology* 1986;28:512–27

8. Zieger M, Dörr U, Schulz RD. Pediatric spinal sonography. Part II: Malformations and mass lesions. *Pediatr Radiol* 1988;18:105–11

9. Kawahara H, Andou Y, Takashima S, *et al*. Normal development of the spinal cord in neonates and infants seen on ultrasonography. *Neuroradiology* 1987;29:50–2

10. Beek FJA, Bax KMA, Mali WPTM. Sonography of the coccyx in newborns and infants. *J Ultrasound Med* 1994;13:629–34

11. St. Amour TE, Rubin JM, Dohrmann GJ. The central canal of the spinal cord: ultrasonic identification. *Radiology* 1984;152:767–9

12. St. Amour TE, Rubin JM, Dohrmann GJ. Letter to editor. *Radiology* 1985;155:536

13. Nelson MD Jr, Sedler JA, Gilles GH. Spinal cord central echo complex: histoanatomic correlation. *Radiology* 1989;170:479–81

14. Resjö IM, Harwood-Nash DC, Fitz CR, *et al*. Normal cord in infants and children examined with computed tomographic metrizamide myelography. *Radiology* 1979;130:691–6

15. Quencer RM, Montalvo BM. Normal intraoperative spinal sonography. *Am J Radiol* 1984;143:1301–5

16. Schumacher R, Kroll B, Schwarz M, *et al*. M-mode sonography of the caudal spinal cord in patients with meningomyelocele; work in progress. *Radiology* 1992;184:263–5

17. Wilson DA, Prince JR. MR imaging determination of the location of normal conus medullaris throughout childhood. *Am J Child* 1989;152: 1029–32

18. DiPietro MA. The conus medullaris: normal US findings throughout childhood. *Radiology* 1993;188: 149–53

19. Wolf S, Schneble F, Troger J. The conus medullaris: time of ascendence to normal level. *Pediatr Radiol* 1992;22:590–2

20. Koroshetz AM, Taveras JM. Anatomy of the vertebrae and spinal cord. In Taveras JM, ed. *Radiology-Diagnosis-Imaging-Intervention*. Philadelphia: J.B. Lippincott Co, 1986:5

21. Beek FJA, van Leeuwen MS, Bax NMA, *et al*. A method for sonographic counting of the lower vertebral bodies in newborns and infants. *Am J Neuroradiol* 1994;15:445–9

22. Reigel DH. Tethered spinal cord. *Concepts Pediatr Neurosurg* 1983;4:142–64

23. Chapman PH. Congenital intraspinal lipomas: anatomic considerations and surgical treatment. *Child's Brain* 1982;9:37–47

24. Emery JL, Lendon RG. Lipomas of the cauda equina and other fatty tumours related to neuro-spinal dysraphism. *Dev Med Child Neurol Suppl* 1969; 20:62–70

25. Lhowe D, Ehrlich MG, Chapman PH, *et al*. Congenital intraspinal lipomas: clinical presentation and response to treatment. *J Pediatr Orthop* 1987;7: 531–7

26. Naidich TP, McLone DG, Mutluer S. A new understanding of dorsal dysraphism with lipoma (lipomyeloschisis): radiologic evaluation and surgical correction. *Am J Radiol* 1983;140:1065–78

27. Brunelle F, Sebag G, Baraton J, *et al*. Lumbar spinal cord motion measurement with phase-contrast MR imaging in normal children and in children with spinal lipomas. *Pediatr Radiol* 1996;26:265–70

28. Raghavendra BN, Epstein FJ, Pinto RS, *et al*. The tethered spinal cord: diagnosis by high-resolution real-time ultrasound. *Radiology* 1983;149:123–8

29. Yamada S, Zinke DE, Sanders D. Pathophysiology of the 'tethered cord syndrome'. *J Neurosurg* 1981;54: 494–503

30. Kriss VM, Kriss TC, Babcock DS. The ventriculus terminalis of the spinal cord in the neonate: a normal variant on sonography. *Am J Radiol* 1995;165:1491–3

31. Rypens F, Avni EF, Matos C, *et al*. Atypical and equivocal sonographic features of the spinal cord in neonates. *Pediatr Radiol* 1995;25:429–32

32. Avni EF, Matos C, Grassart A, *et al*. Sinus pilonidaux neonatals et echographie medullaire de depistage: resultats preliminaires. *Pediatrie* 1991;46:607–11

33. Nelson MD Jr, Bracchi M, Naidich TP, *et al*. The natural history of repaired myelomeningocele. *RadioGraphics* 1988;8:695–706

34. Hoffman HJ, Neill J, Crone KR, *et al*. Hydrosyringomyelia and its management in childhood. *Neurosurgery* 1987;21:347–51

35. Hoffman HJ, Taecholarn C, Hendrick EB, et al. Management of lipomyelomeningoceles: experience at the Hospital for Sick Children, Toronto. J Neurosurg 1985;62:1–8

36. Schlesinger AE, Naidich TP, Quencer RM. Concurrent hydromyelia and diastematomyelia. Am J Neuroradiol 1986;7:473–7

37. Brühl K, Schwarz M, Schumacher R, et al. Congenital diastematomyelia in the upper thoracic spine. Diagnostic comparison of CT, CT-myelography, MRI and US. Neurosurg Rev 1990;13:77–82

38. Raghavendra BN, Epstein FJ, Pinto RS, et al. Sonographic diagnosis of diastematomyelia. J Ultrasound Med 1988;7:111–13

39. Glasier CM, Chadduck WM, Leithiser RE Jr, et al. Screening spinal ultrasound in newborns with neural tube defects. J Ultrasound Med 1990;9:339–43

40. Venes JL, Stevens EA. Surgical pathology in tethered cord secondary to myelomeningocele repair. Concepts Pediatr Neurosurg 1983;4:165–85

41. Quencer RM, Montalvo BM, Naidich TP, et al. Intraoperative sonography in spinal dysraphism and syringohydromyelia. Am J Radiol 1987;148:1005–13

42. Jacobs NM, Grant EG, Dagi TF, et al. Ultrasound identification of neural elements in myelomeningocele. J Clin Ultrasound 1984;12:51–3

43. Cramer BC, Jequier S, O'Gorman AM. Sonography of the neonatal craniocervical junction. Am J Radiol 1986;147:133–9

44. Storrs BB, Reid BS, Walker ML. Ultrasound evaluation of the Chiari II malformation in infants. Concepts Pediatr Neurosurg 1985;6:172–80

45. DiPietro MA, Venes JL. Intraoperative sonography of Arnold-Chiari malformations. In Rubin JM, Chandler WF, eds. Ultrasound in Neurosurgery, New York: Raven Press, 1990:183–99

46. DiPietro MA, Venes JL, Rubin JM. Arnold-Chiari II malformation: intraoperative real-time sonography. Radiology 1987;164:799–804

47. Powell KR, Cherry JD, Hougen TJ, et al. A prospective search for congenital dermal abnormalities of the craniospinal axis. J Pediatr 1975;87:744–50

48. Storrs BB, Walker ML. Sacral dermal sinus – occult sacral masses discovered by routine ultrasound. Concepts Pediatr Neurosurg 1987;7:172–8

49. Nelson MD Jr, Segall HD, Gwinn JL. Sonography in newborns with cutaneous manifestations of spinal abnormalities. Am Fam Physician 1989;40:198–203

50. Hall DE, Udvarhelyi GB, Altman J. Lumbosacral skin lesions as markers of occult spinal dysraphism. J Am Med Assoc 1981;246:2606–8

51. Radkowski MA, Byrd SE, McLone DG. Clinical and sonographic correlation of sacrococcygeal dimples. Presented at the 33rd Annual Meeting of the Society for Pediatric Radiology, April 1990

52. Korsvik HE, Keller MS. Sonography of occult dysraphism in neonates and infants with MR imaging correlation. RadioGraphics 1992;12:297–306

53. Albright AL, Gartner JC, Wiener ES. Lumbar cutaneous hemangiomas as indicators of tethered spinal cords. Pediatrics 1989;83:977–80

54. Higginbottom MC, Jones KL, James HE, et al. Aplasia cutis congenita: a cutaneous marker of occult spinal dysraphism. J Pediatr 1980;96:687–9

55. Appignani BA, Jaramillo D, Barnes PD, et al. Dysraphic myelodysplasias associated with urogenital and anorectal anomalies: prevalence and types seen with MR imaging. Am J Radiol 1994;163:1199–203

56. Beek FJA, Boemers TML, Witkamp TD, et al. Spine evaluation in children with anorectal malformations. Pediatr Radiol 1995;25:S28–32

57. Carson JA, Barnes PD, Tunell WP, et al. Imperforate anus: the neurologic implication of sacral abnormalities. J Pediatr Surg 1984;19:838–42

58. Karrer FM, Flannery AM, Nelson MD Jr, et al. anorectal malformations: evaluation of associated spinal dysraphic syndromes. J Pediatr Surg 1988;23:45–8

59. McHugh K, Dudley NE, Tam P. Pre-operative MRI of anorectal anomalies in the newborn period. Pediatr Radiol 1995;25:S33–6

60. Tunell WP, Austin JC, Barnes PD, et al. Neuroradiologic evaluation of sacral abnormalities in imperforate anus complex. J Pediatr Surg 1987;22:58–61

61. Long FR, Hunter JV, Mahboubi S, et al. Tethered cord and associated vertebral anomalies in children and infants with imperforate anus: evaluation with MR imaging and plain radiography. Radiology 1996;200:377–82

62. Currarino G, Coln D, Votteler T. Triad of anorectal, sacral and presacral anomalies. Am J Radiol 1981;137:395–8

63. Kirks DR, Merten DF, Filston HC, et al. The Currarino triad: complex of anorectal malformation, sacral bony abnormality, and prescral mass. Pediatr Radiol 1984;14:220–5

64. Yates VD, Wilroy RS, Whitington GL, et al. Anterior sacral defects: an autosomal dominantly inherited condition. J Pediatr 1983;102:239–42

65. Anderson FM. occult spinal dysraphism: a series of 73 cases. Pediatrics 1975;55:826–35

# Index